꧁꧂꧁꧂꧁꧂꧁꧂꧁꧂꧁꧂꧁꧂꧁꧂꧁꧂꧁꧂꧁꧂꧁꧂꧁꧂

Ten Books of Surgery

꧁꧂꧁꧂꧁꧂꧁꧂꧁꧂꧁꧂꧁꧂꧁꧂꧁꧂꧁꧂꧁꧂꧁꧂꧁꧂

Ten Books of Surgery

with
The Magazine of the Instruments Necessary for It

By

AMBROISE PARÉ

Translated by

ROBERT WHITE LINKER

and

NATHAN WOMACK

UNIVERSITY OF GEORGIA PRESS

ATHENS

Paperback edition, 2010
© 1969 by the University of Georgia Press
Athens, Georgia 30602
www.ugapress.org
Printed digitally in the United States of America

The Library of Congress has cataloged the
hardcover edition of this book as follows:

Library of Congress Cataloging-in-Publication Data

Paré, Ambroise, 1510?-1590.
    Ten books of surgery, with the magazine
of the instruments necessary for it. Translated by
Robert White Linker and Nathan Womack.
    xvi, 264 p. illus. 23 cm.
Translation of Dix livres de la chirurgie.
    1. Surgery —Early works to 1800. I. Title.
RD30 .P3613
617'.1   68-25355

Paperback ISBN-13: 978-0-8203-3548-3
ISBN-10: 0-8203-3548-7

Contents

To

Dorothy Insley Linker
and
Margaret Richardson Womack

SHORT TITLE LIST OF PARE'S WORKS

1. *La Méthode de traicter les playes,* 1545
2. *La Maniere de traicter les playes,* 1551
3. *Briefve collection de l'administration anatomique,* 1549
4. *Anatomie universelle du corps humain,* 1561
5. *La Méthode curative des playes de la teste,* 1561
6. *Dix livres de la chirurgie,* 1564
7. *Traicté de la peste . . . verolle . . . rougeolle . . . lepre,* 1568
8. *Cinq livres de chirurgie,* 1572
9. *Deux livres de chirurgie,* 1573
10. *Responce de M. Ambroise Paré . . . aux calomnies,* 1575(?)
11. *Les Oeuvres de M. Ambroise Paré,* 1575
12. *Discours de la mumie, de la licorne,* 1582
13. *Replique d'Ambroise Paré,* 1584
14. [Sonnet] to M. J. Guillemeau, 1585
15. [Poem] "A Jaques Guillemeau", 1586

ERRATA

These errors were omitted from the final page proof corrections before the printing of the text of the book.

Page 11, footnote—*locus* should read *locis*.

P. 35, line 30—climeni: *clymenon*.

P. 45, l. 33; p. 46, l. 4, p. 47, l. 2; p. 56, l. 24—of storax, of calamite: *of cane storax*.

P. 46, l. 1—mosch. gra.: *musk grains*.

P. 47, l. 6—suffitus: *perfume*.

P. 56, l. 13—fermento: *yeast;* l. 14—ruthacei: *rue;* l. 28—fermenti acris: *sharp yeast;* l. 29—aqua vini: *water of wine;* l. 29-30—ignem non experti: *not tried by fire.*

P. 84, l. 4—descriptione filagri: *Philagrius's description.*

P. 93, l. 19—rub. torref.: *torrified rhubarb.*

P. 94, l. 20—setaceum: *silk cloth.*

P. 98, l. 17—ireatum: *with iris.*

P. 115, l. 1; p. 233, l. 3—smallpox: *the pox.*

P. 118, l. 17—quinquenerviae: *lesser plantain.*

P. 118, l. 20; p. 182, l. 10—omnium capillarium recentium: *all fresh maidenhair ferns.*

P. 130, l. 34—risatarum: *rockets.*

P. 155, footnote—Pocis: *Locis.*

P. 161. l. 37—mucores: *lees.*

P. 181, l. 36; p. 186, l. 6—violariae: *violet leaves.*

P. 182, l. 8; p. 184, l. 16; p. 186, l. 8; p. 215, l. 14—gammis: *dog's grass.*

P. 182, l. 10—ominum (omnium) capill.: *of all maidenhair ferns.*

P. 182, l. 35—nucleorum: *kernels of.*

P. 187, l. 4—cimini: *cumin.*

Preface

SEVERAL years ago through the kindly interests of the late Mr. Henry Schuman and the enthusiasm of Miss Myrl Ebert, Librarian of the University of North Carolina School of Medicine, that library acquired a copy of *Dix livres de la chirurgie* by Ambroise Paré. Our interest in this little volume was immediate and a translation was undertaken.

The book bears the imprint of Jean le Royer, royal engraver and printer, with the date 1564. The privilege at the end of the book is dated 1559 and the date of printing is given as February 1563. The volume is octavo in size and distributed throughout are several woodcuts, some colored by hand, to illustrate certain instruments mentioned by Paré. The latter part of the book contains woodcuts that serve to illustrate "le magasin des instruments necessaires a icelle."

This is the first English translation of *Dix livres*. There are several reasons for this, perhaps the most cogent being the fact that most of the material in it was subsequently incorporated into Paré's well-known *Oeuvres* which was published in 1575. Another possible reason is the dearth of copies of *Dix livres*. Miss Janet Doe in her excellent bibliography* gives the location of fourteen known copies. Our copy, which was obtained from a book shop in France, is not listed by her.

The translation has not been easy. Paré was a man of little formal education and he wrote in the vernacular of the period. Many times his sentences are exceedingly long, the construction tedious, and on some occasions his grammar questionable. At other times, however, his prose is vivid.

In a book of this type there is always a conflict as to what kind of translation is best—what the author meant or what the author said. In a medical treatise there is a temptation to substitute modern terms in place of the older usages, thereby making the work somewhat anachronistic. This we have chosen not to do

---

*Janet Doe, *A Bibliography of the Works of Ambroise Paré: Premier Chirurgien & Conseiller du Roy* (University of Chicago Press, 1937).

with the full realization that it would make reading more difficult. We have felt that the substitution of present day terminology would do damage to Paré's characteristic style. Punctuation, quite different in the sixteenth century, has been partly modernized. On the other hand, many awkward constructions have not been altered and even grammatical errors have been allowed to remain in order to maintain the style of the vernacular language in which Paré wrote.

BIOGRAPHICAL SKETCH OF PARE*

Ambroise Paré was born in Laval, Maine, in 1517, or perhaps in 1516, old style. Little is actually known of his early life, in spite of the fact that numerous details have been given by a number of biographers without any verifiable basis. Just one illustration: it has been stated that his parents were Huguenots before the time of either Luther or Calvin. It is known that Paré's father was a cabinet-maker. The next known fact is that Paré was in Angers in 1525, and later in Vitré with his brother Jehan, a surgeon.

Paré started working under a barber and moved to Paris in about 1532. At a later date he reported that he had studied surgery for nine or ten years, and that he was at the Hotel Dieu for three years. This ancient institution, which was in poor condition in the sixteenth century, gave Paré opportunities to operate, to study diseases, and to perform dissections on cadavers. This experience helped him later to be admitted by examination to the rank of master barber-surgeon. In addition to acquiring practical experience, Paré also became acquainted with the work of Gui de Chauliac whom he called Guidon.

Renewal of war between François I and Emperor Charles V in 1536 gave Paré his first experience with war and gunshot wounds. All he had known previously about such wounds he had read in Giovanni da Vigo. At first Paré used the usual prescribed remedies but his experiences led him later to experimentation and change. During this war, he had served as surgeon to the Marshal de Montjean, commander of the French infantry, but after the death of the Marshal, Paré refused the offer of the new commander to stay with him and returned to Paris. He took with him at least three new treatments: oil of puppies,

*For a more extensive biography, see J. F. Malgaigne, *Surgery and Ambroise Paré*, translated from the French and edited by Wallace B. Hamby, M.D. (University of Oklahoma Press, 1965).

the secret of a surgeon at Turin, which he had secured by entreaty and gifts; crushed onions for burns, learned from an old woman in Turin; and a new method of treating paraphimosis, learned from an old surgeon of Milan.

He remained in Paris from 1539 to 1543, during which time he married the daughter of a minor official. Renewal of the war in 1543 found him in Perpignan, in the service of M. de Rohan of Brittany. Returning to Paris the next year, Paré discussed his experiences with Jacques du Bois, professor of surgery, who encouraged him to make public his ideas. The result was the publication of Paré's first book, *La Methode de traicter les playes*, printed in 1545 by Vivant Gaulterot, printer of the University of Paris. It was not, as has been said, "the first scientifice book written in French." It was published amid a considerable number of French translations of such writers as Giovanni da Vigo, Hippocrates, Galen, and Paul of Aegina.

Attendant upon this flow of translations was a strong reaction from the medical Faculté in Paris, not only against the translations, but against the general efforts of barbers and surgeons to raise their status. The physicians saw these efforts as a threat to their own prestige and power. The surgeons of the Confraternity of St. Côme might have been expected to lead these efforts, but it was the barbers who did most to raise the level of practice in both anatomy and surgery. It should not be omitted here that in the same year, 1545, Estienne de la Rivière, a surgeon, won a suit for plagiarism against Charles Estienne, professor of medicine.

After another brief service with the army, Paré turned his attention to a more detailed study of anatomy. Aided in this by encouragement from Jacques du Bois, and by dissections with his friend, master barber-surgeon Thierry de Héry, and Jean Colombier, Paré published in 1549 his *Briefve collection de l'administration anatomique*, which included a section on obstetrics. This book met the need for a non-Latin manual for the barber-surgeon, and for the first time since the ancients it presented a description of podalic version. Paré used translations of Galen and of Charles Estienne's *De dissectione* as references.

More military action gained Paré the friendship of the future king of Navarre who recommended him to the king of France. As a result, Paré was named surgeon-in-ordinary to Henri II in 1552.

During the siege of Metz in 1552 by imperial forces, Paré was sent through the besiegers' lines into the town. He was warmly received, not only because of his reputation, but especially because of the extreme need for his services. After the siege failed, Paré was sent to Hesdin, which had surrendered, and was taken prisoner. He exchanged his fine clothing to escape recognition but finally admitted he was a surgeon. The Duke of Savoy, head of the victors, wanted him to enter his service or be sent to the galleys. Luckily the governor of Gravelines gave him his freedom. Henri II had offered to pay ransom for Paré, but since payment was not necessary the king gave Paré a large sum of money instead.

The next important event in Paré's life was his admission as surgeon to the one-time Confraternity of St. Côme, now a college of the University of Paris. Statutes required that a candidate be examined in Latin, which Paré tells us he did not know. However, he was quickly passed through the standard grades and made master on December 18, 1554. The Faculté of physicians kept quiet, at least for the time being.

Peace between king and emperor was finally made. Henri II did not long survive it, dying in 1559 from an injury received in a tournament. Paré retained his place as surgeon to François II during that monarch's brief eighteen-months reign. The following reign of Charles IX was marred by civil war against the Huguenots. Paré, again royal surgeon, followed the king in several campaigns.

In 1561 Paré published his *Anatomie universelle du corps humain*. While the *Fabrica* of Vesalius had gone through several Latin editions, the barber-surgeon, the common surgical practitioner, was unfamiliar with Latin. In 1559 a French translation of Vesalius appeared. From this translation Paré borrowed considerably for his *Anatomie*, but gave full credit to Vesalius. He also made use of his own experiences, which were extensive. While the *Anatomie* was in no sense equal to that of Vesalius in detail and in clarity, it had tremendous popular appeal and was used extensively in the practice of surgery for over half a century.

After the publication of *Dix livres* in 1564, Paré spent two years traveling throughout the provinces with the king. During the trip, Paré was bitten by a viper at Montpellier, but promptly cured himself. At this time many parts of the country were affected by outbreaks of the plague, and Paré fell victim but escaped with only a large scar. A considerable outbreak of smallpox also occurred; Paré, ever ready to observe and to profit by experience, produced a *Traicté de la peste . . . verolle . . . rougeolle . . . lepre* in 1568. One of Paré's prescriptions, which approved the use of antimony, included in this volume aroused the hostility of the Faculté. Paré later omitted it from his complete works.

Paré's reputation continued to grow. By 1570 Dalechamps, in his *Chirurgie française*, had added Paré to the list of great authorities of antiquity and the Moslem world. This was great tribute indeed, especially as the year before Lepaulmier, a member of the Faculté, had blamed Paré for the great number of deaths which had occurred during the siege of Rouen. The siege had been marked by excessive deaths from putrefaction and gangrene, and the king had asked Paré for an explanation which he had given in the first part of the *Dix livres* in 1564. Paré countered Lepaulmier's charge with a defense of his treatment of gunshot wounds in *Cinq livres de chirurgie*, which was published in 1572. Also included in this volume was a discussion of tumors which were generally considered to be in the province of physicians. The success of *Cinq livres* spoiled interest in Gourmelen's *Surgical synopsis* and increased the hostility of the Faculté toward Paré.

In 1573 Paré, whose first wife had died, married for the second time. The same year he published his *Deux livres de chirurgie*, which contained a considerable discussion of generation and material on monsters. The next year Henri III succeeded Charles IX, and Paré not only remained premier-surgeon to the new king but was advanced to the rank of *valet-de-chambre* and *conseiller*.

The year 1575 saw the appearance of the first folio edition of Paré's complete works, *Les Oeuvres de M. Ambroise Paré, conseiller et premier chirurgien du roi*. Gourmelen, who had been elected dean of the Faculté the previous year, took advantage of an old law to try to even an old score. Involved was Faculté approval of a medical work before publication and Paré's book was brought before Parlement in a lawsuit. Among objections, other than Gourmelen's personal bias, was the fact that the book intruded on the field of the physician and was written in French rather than Latin. Even the surgeons of the College of St. Côme did not approve of Paré's writing about professional matters in the vernacular. None of these objections stopped the publication of *Oeuvres*, but the troubles continued between the Faculté and the surgeons and Paré. In the second edition of the *Oeuvres* in 1579, Paré answered several of the attacks made against him.

Paré next turned his attention to a denunciation of the use of mummy and of the unicorn's horn, long fabled as an antidote for all poisons and highly treasured by kings. An answer, approved by the Faculté, to Paré's latest breach of medical tradition was immediately forthcoming. He was accused of stepping out of his field to attack physicians and apothecaries. During the ensuing years Paré was frequently attacked by Gourmelen, and in the fourth edition of the *Oeuvres*, Paré again answered these accusations.

Paré's last years were spent rather quietly, in spite of the civil wars raging throughout France. Paris, where he was living, was besieged in 1589 by Henri III and again in 1590 by Henri IV. Paré died on August 29, four months after the siege was lifted.

It is generally stated that Paré made three great contributions to surgery: the use of bland ointments rather than hot oil in the treatment of gunshot wounds, podalic version, and the preliminary ligation of major vessels in amputation. Preliminary ligation is described for the first time in *Dix livres*. The use of bland ointments for gunshot wounds was included in his first volume and is discussed again in considerable detail in *Dix livres*. These were important contributions to the practice of surgery at that time and in no sense should one denigrate them. On the other hand, they themselves are hardly adequate to catapult this relatively obscure barber-surgeon to a position of surgeon and adviser to kings, respected by the poor and great alike, and to a position of dominance in surgery that was to last for centuries. We must therefore look for something else.

Paré possessed inordinate intellectual and physical courage. Such was necessary for independent thinking in medicine in France at that time. This was a period of established dogma and of superstition. Astrology was practiced often by the best minds and even Paré on occasion brought it into use. Nevertheless, where facts justified he willingly broke with tradition; thus in his discussion of the treatment of hemorrhage by the cauterization of vessels he had this to say:

"I counsel the young surgeon to abandon this miserable manner of burning and butchering, admonishing him not to say any more, 'I have seen it in the book of the ancient practitioners, I have seen it done by my old fathers and masters, following whose practice I can in no way fail.' This I grant you if you wish to listen to your good master Galen in the book referred to above, and those like him, but if you wish to stop at your father and masters in order to have prescriptioners of time and license of ill-doing, wishing always to persevere in it, such as one does to a certain degree ordinarily in all things, you will render account of it before GOD and not before your father or your good practitioner masters, who treat men in so cruel a fashion."

He saw the intellectual and moral deficit of many of the barber-surgeons of the period, and since he was one of them, sought to elevate their position by education and example. Most of his surgical knowledge had been acquired by observation and experience and he recommended this to others. In discussing his method of the ligation of blood vessels he states: "You may find this method of practicing rather obscure and difficult to understand, but you must consider that it is a very difficult thing to put manual surgery clearly and entirely in writing, for it is rather to be learned by imagination and by seeing good and experienced masters perform, if you have the means or, indeed, to try it on dead bodies as I have done many times."

He frequently performed an autopsy to determine the cause of death. While realizing the value of a dry wound he recognized the fact that this could rarely be obtained with the type of gunshot wound that he so frequently was called upon to treat. Familiar with the hazard of a spreading, deep infection he believed that contused wounds should be led to suppuration and here he seeks support from Galen. "Galen quotes Hippocrates, saying, if the flesh is contused, bruised or beaten by some dart or in other manner, that it must be medicated in such a way that it suppurates the soonest possible." He advocated the drainage of such wounds by tents and setons, and the surgeon was admonished not to pack his wounds too tight—not to use setons or tents that were too large as they prevented adequate drainage. After good drainage had been established he recommended the use of canulae made of gold or silver or lead. He stressed the need for the removal of foreign bodies from such wounds and paid considerable attention to the use of the proper instrument in such a maneuver.

His power of observation is well illustrated in his description of the meticulous care that must be used in splinting fractures. He advocated early mobilization of fractures as soon as the callus would permit; and in amputations, where possible, the site was related to the function of an artificial limb. The artificial limbs depicted in this book are by no means all of his design. With the aid of an artificial limb maker he had an opportunity to combine his knowledge of anatomy and surgery with good mechanics.

To Paré surgery required courage:

"For the surgeon with the piteous face
Renders the wound of his patient verminous."

This did not mean a lack of gentleness and concern. It is of interest that one of the reasons that he gives for advocating preliminary ligations of the major vessels in amputations is that it rapidly produces numbness of the extremity and makes the operation less painful.

Although a surgeon to kings, Paré was also a surgeon to the common soldier and to the common man. This was unusual in the sixteenth century because it was commonplace for many physicians to ignore the illnesses of the common people. His rebuke to the physicians is stinging: "You will be able to have the counsel of the learned physician. Still considering that one cannot always get a physician, I have indeed wished to describe for you here some good and approved remedies. . . ." While some of his therapy such as covering the patient with warm manure is not acceptable today, his concluding statement is: "Therefore, it is necessary that the surgeon have always before his eyes that God and nature command him not to leave patients without doing his duty although he may foresee the signs of death, for nature often does what seems to the surgeon to be impossible."

Paré possessed many of the prejudices of the time and by no means was able to break completely with the dogma of the past. However, in *Dix livres* he shows the ability to see, to reason, and to doubt. As such he was a product of the Renaissance as was no other surgeon. As was anticipated, it is in *Dix livres* that we see him as he reaches the best in his performance.

To the Very Christian King

TWELVE years ago it pleased the majesty of the late King Henry, your father, to receive from me a small book in which my mind was indifferently employed in treating the manner of curing well and surely wounds made by blows of arquebuses and of arrows. This treatise seemed (as my judgment can extend itself) sufficient to protect the wounded from such wounds and preserve them from the complications which customarily occur in such disasters, considering that wounds were not so dangerous at that time and did not carry as many pernicious problems as they have done for the past three or four years, to the great regret of the French people, who with very good occasion can detest the first inventor of this damnable instrument. If things had always remained in such a state, I would not have employed a single hour in reviewing the said treatise for fear of being convicted of a useless and superfluous repetition. But since time has brought with it so many difficulties concerning the cure of these evils, increased and augmented by half at least, who is it who will justly criticize me, if to teach the means of this cure and to alienate from us the pestilent malignities of these deadly wounds, I have again taken in hand my first work in order to amplify it with remedies suitable, indeed necessary, for the said wounds, especially when one will recognize the constitution of the time to be similar to or approach the recent years; otherwise one will turn back to practice according to the method that I have written previously. I dedicate it to Your Majesty, Sire. I believe that the most pitiless, indeed the most barbarous, not entirely despoiled of the mantle of humanity would take my labor only in good part, if, though little civilized and taught in our language, they had the means of reading my book. This makes me prejudge that all the subjects of your crown, surmounting by much those of other nations in noble disposition, grace, and civility of mores, will be grateful

1

to me for the fact that in the review of this work of mine, I shall have done so much for them. I know the matter is not of such weight that it can merit the grandeur of your name, in order to appear to the eyes of your subjects and be brought to light under its favor. Still, wishing to enrich it with another furnishing which is solely addressed to you, I have no hesitancy in presenting the whole to Your Majesty.

I remember, Sire, that it was once your pleasure to ask me how it came about that most of the wounded in these late wars died or escaped with very great difficulty indeed from the arquebus wounds that they had received in fighting. Since I did not satisfy you at the time as I should have wished, I have now, in order to content your royal mind on this point, put in the front of this book a rather ample discourse on the occasions that have inevitably led many people to death. I do not have at present other riches with which I may better my present, at least which are proper for you, except a magazine of the instruments serving in surgery. These, in part invented by me, in part taken and drawn from the books of my predecessors, I present to Your Majesty, knowing well how Your Majesty delights in sometimes handling and seeing them, and very humbly entreat Your Majesty to be willing to accept it only as an earnest of a greater work that I am reserving for Your Majesty, and which by means of the grace of God, who alone disposes of the life of men, Your Majesty will hear soon, I hope. The rest of this present treatise consists only of a few additions and precepts of my art; also it is not you only to whom this piece refers (now that I am making it fly under your name), but the young surgeons, who by this addition of mine will be able diligently to provide for the complications and diversify the manner of treating those who in the future may be wounded in your service. May it please God that the number of them may be rare and that your kingdom may flourish in peace so assured that its people may have no occasion to regret our hands. Which in this place I ask of the Lord God with as good heart as I humbly kiss Your Majesty's hands.

Discourse of M. Ambroise Paré

First Surgeon of the King, on the fact that it pleased the majesty of the said lord one day to ask him concerning the matter of arquebusades and of other firearms.

BECAUSE it one day pleased Your Majesty, Sire, that of the Queen your mother, my lord the Prince de la Roche-sur-Yon, and several other princes and great lords to ask me how it came about that in these last wars most of the gentlemen and soldiers wounded by blows of arquebuses and other instruments died without our being able in any way to cure them, or with very great difficulty recovered from their injuries, even though the wounds received by them were of very small appearance and though the surgeons called for their cure employed all their duty and knowledge in it, I have, indeed, dared to put forward this discourse, in part to satisfy the duty of my art and not detract from the highest honor of my profession, which Your Majesty has fully continued to me to this day, and in part to have you understand the reasons which can have caused the death of so many valiant men. Most of these I have seen, to my great regret, end their days piteously without it being possible for me, or for any other more experienced than I, to give them any remedy.

I know that the following discourse will astonish some who rest on their personal opinions and do not explore matters to the bottom of the sack. They will find the first part of my discussion rather strange because, contrary to what for a long time they have had imprinted in their minds, I do not grant them that the cause of the malignity of arquebusades proceeds from the venom or poisoning which their brains dream is carried by the cannon powder, or by the balls steeped and fried in some venomous matter. Yet if their courtesy and patience also can extend so far, they may be willing to weigh the zeal which

3

has moved me to profit the republic. Toward this in the past I have striven to make avail the talent which the singular providence of God has willed to allot to me, and even now I employ myself further in it. If also their patience will use their entire judgment to examine the reasons which I use in this present treatise, I am sure that they will hold my labor agreeable and will exempt it from all calumny, or else that they will be so badly affected with regard to it that even if I addressed myself to them enriched with all the treasures of the ancient philosophers, they would still want to put me in the rank of the most impoverished and ignorant men in the whole world.

In order then to obviate the arguments that the favorers of venom and poisoning mentioned above could put in play, I shall show Your Majesty, Sire, that the offense of the arquebusades does not come from the venom that the powder or the ball carries with itself, and still even less from the combustion or burn that the said ball, heated by the fire put in the powder, makes in the parts that it breaks by its violence. Nevertheless, some try to sustain this concept, alleging for total reasons that formerly a tower full of powder was seen ruined in an instant by a single cannon shot. Similarly, a house covered by thatch was set on fire by the single shot of an arquebus. Furthermore, in the practice of the wounds that fire instruments make, we ordinarily see the orifices and the parts surrounding the said wounds so black that one would say that an actual cautery had passed over them. All of these arguments are so badly supported that their foundation does not merit one's stopping on them and even less taking the answer to your question from them, as I hope to have you understand by the discussion which follows. For after having seen a great number of such wounds, these observed diligently and medicated by great method, I have collected from the ancient philosophers, physicians, and surgeons, information to present to Your Majesty, and with this to withdraw it from the wonder that it had of the frightful death of so many gentlemen and good soldiers.

Now, to enter into the matter and to answer the arguments alleged above, it seems good to me to discuss first whether there is any venom enclosed in cannon powder and, further, if there were any, if it can infect us by its said venom. In order to deduce this point perfectly, I am forced to search the composition of this powder, considering that it is not of simple substance, but compound, and then to pursue the nature of the simples which enter into its composition, their qualities, effects, and operations. As for the simples, it is a quite assured thing that there are only three which compose it, that is, charcoal of willow or of hemp stalks, sulphur, and saltpeter, sometimes also brandy, which ingredients considered separately are exempt from all venom. Since it is thus, the charcoal has no particular quality in itself except a dryness in a subtle substance by means of which it receives the fire as easily as a burnt cloth receives the sparks from a gun. The sulphur, warm and dry in degree, not however excessive, is of more oily and viscid substance yet not as easy to inflame as the charcoal, although it retains the fire very lively when it is seized by it and is extinguished only with great difficulty. Saltpeter is such that many use it in place of salt.

Thus we discover that there is no poison in the nature of these simples, particularly in that of sulphur, which is the most suspect, seeing even that Galen commands, in the ninth book of *Simple Medicaments*, to have those drink it who are bitten by venomous beasts and to apply it externally to those who have galls. Now as for brandy, it is such a subtle thing that it evaporates and is consumed if one throws it in the air; furthermore, surgeons order it often in drinks and lotions for a greatly similar remedy. This causes me to say that the whole composition is exempt from venom since its ingredients are so sound, each in its place, that the German horsemen injured by some arquebusade make no difficulty of dissolving in wine two charges of cannon powder and swallowing them, hoping by this means to recover their health and obviate the complications which happen to their wounds, which I do not approve. But what does it serve me to allege a foreign example since I have seen many French soldiers by I know not what gaiety of heart who, wishing to show themselves to be good companions, swallow a rather good quantity of it without, however, receiving any trouble from it? Others, wounded in a place in their body, apply some of it on their ulcers to dry them and find themselves very well for it.

As for those who say it is not the powder but the bullet that finely pierced in many places and filled with venom or steeped, fried, and mixed in some poison, causes this dangerous excess, I can answer them, without belaboring myself much, that the fire put in the powder would purify the venom of the ball, if there were any in it. To say also that it is the combustion of the bullet that causes the danger I cannot understand, seeing that the balls, composed ordinarily of lead, could not stand so extreme heat without melting and dissolving fully. However, we see them pass through a harness and penetrate the body through and through and still remain entire. Further, we observe when one fires them against a stone or some other solid material that they can in the same instant be handled by us and held in the hand without their giving off notable or ardent heat, although the touching and collision of these with the stone ought to increase their warmth, if any were there. What is more, if one fires any ball into a sack full of cannon powder, it in no way catches fire. Therefore, I dare boldly to say and assure that when fire is put to a powder stored in some tower or other place, that this is done not by the fire nor the ball themselves but by the attrition of this striking against the stone of the said tower and making sparks of fire come from it which fall into the powder, no more nor less than in the wick of the gun we see some sparks fall by the collision of the iron and the flint. We are to judge the same of the thatch coverings, which are not kindled by the heat accompanying the bullet but rather by some cloth, wadding, or other such material attached to the ball. What makes me firmer in the assurance of my saying is that if we wish to fire a ball of wax carrying no fire with itself (for otherwise it would melt), yet will it pierce a wood of the thickness of half a finger, a sufficiently valid argument to show that bullets cannot be heated so that they will cauterize and burn as some have esteemed.

And to explain the blackness which is ordinarily found in the orifices of wounds and the nearby parts, I say this accident does not come by reason of some fire accompanying the ball but because of the great contusion that it makes, and because also the air is not able to enter the body except by an unbelievable force and violence because of the smallness and narrow roundness of the wound, rendering it quite black and the parts around quite livid. If one wished to question such wounded men, I believe that they would be sufficient witness of what I say because they are not so quickly struck that at the same instant it did not seem to them that a beam or other similar weight had fallen on the injured part, in which also they feel an aggravating pain, a numbness, and a sleepiness which dissipates and sometimes extinguishes the natural warmth, with the spirits which are contained in it, whence most often ensue gangrene and mortification of the part, indeed sometimes of the entire body.

Although these reasons show rather evidently that there is no venom in cannon powder nor any fire carried by the bullet, still it is that many, throwing themselves on natural philosophy, maintain quite the contrary and, to prevail over me in this opinion, say that cannon shots are entirely similar to the blows of thunder and thunderbolts which the broken clouds in the middle region of the air precipitate onto the earth. From this simile, they infer and conclude that there is fire and venom in the bullet coming out of the mouth of the cannon. I know, thank God, that the thunderbolt, formed from a dense and thick exhalation by means of the vapor which is conjoined to it, never shatters the cloud to hurl itself here below that it does not drag with itself some fire, now thinner, again thicker, according to the diversity of the matter of which the exhalation is composed; for Seneca writes in the second book of his *Natural Questions*, chapter forty-ninth, that there are only three kinds of thunderbolts, all differing from each other according to the quantity and sort of their inflammation, the one which, because of its more subtle and tenuous matter, pierces only and penetrates, as in making a hole, the objects that it strikes; the next which by its violence breaks and dissipates the same things because its matter is more compact and turbulent as a storm; and the third, which composed of a more terrestrial matter, burns with obvious evidence of its heat. I know further that the thunderbolt is of a fetid and pestilent nature for the reason that its dense and viscid matter when burned gives up such a stinking odor that the animals, accustomed to lodge in their caverns and dens, are constrained to abandon them if perchance the thunderbolt has fallen there, not being able to endure the fetid stench of this poison.

Thus it is that, for these reasons, I will not agree that cannon shots are accompanied by poison and fire, as are thunderbolts, for although they resemble each other in some ways, it is not, however, in their substance and matter but rather in the manner they have of breaking, crushing, and dissipating the objects they encounter, that is, thunderbolts by their fire and by the stone sometimes engendered in this, and cannon shots by the violently pushed air which, guiding a ball, makes a similar disaster. But if I were convinced by stronger arguments, as far as admitting thunderbolts and cannon to be of similar substance, still I should not be forced to say that cannonades and arquebusades carry fire with themselves, considering that among the thunderbolts there are some (as Pliny says in the second book of his *History*, chapter fifty-first) which, composed of marvelously dry matter, dissipate everything they encounter without however burning it in any way. Others are of more humid nature, which likewise do not burn but blacken exceedingly; and some of a much clearer and diaphanous matter, the nature of which is so marvelous that one cannot doubt (as Seneca has well said) that there is not in them some divine virtue, in that they subtly melt gold and silver, without involving the wallets and purses in any way. They melt a sword, the scabbard remaining in its entirety. They cause the iron of a pike to distil without the wood's becoming warm. They spill the wine of casks without making any opening in them or burning them. Accordingly, I could assure, and without any prejudice, that the thunderbolts which only break and dissipate without in any way burning and which leave some extraordinary effects are similar in substance to cannonades, but not those which at the same time carry both flame and fire.

In order to confirm my saying, I shall be content with the example of a soldier from whose thigh I remember that I drew a bullet which, enveloped by the taffeta of his breeches, had made him a deep wound, yet I drew it from him with the same taffeta without its being in any way involved or burned. What is more, I have seen many men who, without being struck or in any way touched even in their apparel, have received such stunning from the cannonades passing near them that their members have become completely black and livid from it, then soon after have been gangrened and mortified, from which finally they died. These effects are similar to those of the thunderbolt. Yet there is in them no fire or venom, which makes me boldly conclude that there is no poison in the ordinary artifice of powder.

Then, since the disaster has been common to all those who have been wounded in these last wars, and that it is not by fire or by venom that so many valiant men have died, to what cause will we be able to impute this misfortune? I am at the place, Sire, where I hope presently to have Your Majesty hear it, in order that Your Majesty may be completely satisfied. Those who have spent their life and study in the secrets of natural philosophy have left us of it, one among others for authentic and approved for all time; that is, that the elements so agree with each other that they are transmuted the one into the other, so that not only their first qualities, which are heat, cold, dryness, and humidity, but also their substances are changed by rarefaction or condensation of itself. Thus fire is converted ordinarily into air, air into water, water into earth and, to the opposite, earth into water, water into air, and air into fire. This we see by the eye and experience in the copper whistles which the Germans bring us, made in the form of a ball which, filled with water and having only a small hole in the middle of its spherical form, receives the transmutation of its water into air by the action of the fire when placed near the ball and pushes the said air out with violence, making it rustle impetuously until it has all gone out. The like can be recognized in chestnuts and marrons when one throws them in the fire without having cracked them. For then the aqueous humidity which is contained in them is changed into air by the action of the fire, and the air, wishing to come out, bursts the marron, because not finding an opening it is constrained to make one by violence. I dare say and affirm as much for the materials contained in cannon powder which, by means of fire, are converted into a great quantity of air which, not being able to be contained in the place where the material was before its transmutation, is forced to issue forth with an unbelievable violence, by means of which it pushes and moves the bullet with itself, which tears, crushes, and breaks everything it encounters. What is more, it drives before itself a wind so rarified and so violently agitated that the bodies are sooner seized by it than by the bullet, although the thing be not discovered by the sight. Quite often, the action is made by this wind alone without the ball's giving its blow, indeed as far as breaking the bones without manifest division of the flesh. This we have already said to be common to the thunderbolt. We experience the same in the said powder when, being enclosed in mines and converted into wind by the fire that one puts in it, it overthrows piles of earth as large as mountains. One has seen this year in your town of Paris a small quantity of powder, freshly made in the arsenal, cause so

9

great a tempest that it made almost all the town tremble, tumbled to the ground all the nearby houses, and unroofed and dewindowed those which were more sheltered from its fury. Briefly, like a crashing thunderbolt, it overthrew here and there some half-dead men. From some, it took away the sight, from others the hearing, and left others no less torn in their poor members than if four horses had quartered them, and this solely by the agitation of the air, into the substance of which the powder was converted. This, according to the quantity and quality of its material, according also to its movement, more or less strong, has caused marvelous events in our provinces wholly similar to those that winds make when enclosed beneath a non-perspirable earth which, wishing to come out, blow with such a strong agitation that they make all the said earth tremble, raising and lowering it, now here, now there, demolishing it, and transporting it from one place to another, as the towns of Megara and Aegina, anciently very celebrated in the land of Greece, yet destroyed by earthquakes, can testify for us. I forego examining (as serving little to our purpose) I know not what loudly blowing rumors and murmurs which the windy matter contained in caverns and subterranean places excites most often, according to the quantity of its matter and the form of the said caverns, as far as representing assaults of towns, bellowing of bulls, and roarings of frightful lions, which however show great similitude with the horrible sounds of artillery. But someone will say these things have been at all times and were no less ordinary in the past than they are at present, and that it is folly for me to allege them for efficient causes of the death of so many men. This I would confess to him with good heart, if it were so that I should present them for such, but seeing that by these I wish only to compare the violence of cannon with that of thunderbolts and movements of the earth, his calumny will not be valid where I am concerned, rather will it be entirely refuted if he is willing to lend his ear to the deduction into which I enter presently in order to determine the principal cause of this death.

In the number of things necessary to our life, there is nothing which can alter us more than the air, which continually willing and unwillingly we breathe in by the conduits which nature has delegated to doing this, such as the mouth, the nose, and generally the openings of the skin, and of the

10

arteries which are adherent to it. This we do in drinking, eating, waking, sleeping, and performing every other natural, vital, and animal action. Thus it is that air inspired in the lungs, the heart, and universally in all the parts of the body in order to refresh them and sometimes to nourish them causes man to be unable to live a single minute without its inspiration. As a result of this beneficient effect, the physician Hippocrates* has truly said that the air has something or other divine in itself because, blowing through the universal world, it encompasses every day all the things contained in it, nourishes them miraculously, sustains them firmly, and holds them in amiable union. The whole agrees with the stars, in which divine providence is infused, which changes the air at its pleasure and gives it power over the mutation of the weather as well as of natural bodies.

Therefore, the philosophers and physicians have expressly commanded paying heed to the situations of the places and to the constitutions of the air when it is a question of keeping the health or of curing maladies, with regard to which the uninterrupted course and change of the said air has very great power, as we can easily recognize by the four seasons of the year. For in summer, the air being warm and dry, our bodies likewise become warm and dry. And in winter the humidity of the air and coldness fill us with the same qualities, in such order, however, and such good disposition of nature that although our temperament seems to change according to the four seasons, still the fact is that we incur no ill, provided that the weathers keep their seasons and qualities exempt from all excess. On the contrary, if the seasons are perverted, in the fashion that the summer is cold, the winter warm, and the others in similar intemperance, this discord brings great perturbation in our bodies as well as in our spirits, which are forced to receive danger from it, for the causes are external, and surround us on all sides. They force us to lodge them in our organs and passages formed by nature, in part to put outside the unnecessary excrements of our nourishment, in part to receive those causes coming from outside, which are the winds, producing diverse effects in us according to the parts of the world whence they proceed. Now since the austral wind is warm and humid, that of the north cold and dry, the oriental clean and pure, that of the west-

---

*De aere, locus et aquis.

southwest nubilous and quite moist with rain, it is a quite assured thing that the air which we breathe in continually partakes wholly and thoroughly of the quality of the wind which by its blowing dominates all the others. Therefore, we must necessarily consider in all diseases and in the complications which occur in them the quality of the winds and the power that they have over our persons. This Hippocrates has learnedly left us in writing in the third book of his *Aphorisms,* saying that our bodies receive great alteration by the south wind which subjects us to all maladies, recognizing humidity for their primary cause, and enfeebles our natural warmth. On the contrary, this is fortified and rendered more vigorous by a cold and dry wind, which likewise renders our spirits more subtle and agile. Also, when Hippocrates compares the temperatures with each other, he concludes that drynesses are without comparison healthier than humidities continued through a long succession of time, because (in his opinion completely according to reason) excessive humidity is the true matter of putrefaction. Experience shows us this in the places where the sea air exercises its tyranny, meat, however fresh it may be, is corrupted and rots in less than a good hour. These things considered, and considering that it is necessary, in order to preserve our bodies in their entirety, that the seasons follow each other step by step in their natural temperature without any excess or extreme difference, there is no doubt that bodies do fall into affection against nature when the seasons pervert their qualities by the bad disposition of the air and of the wind which dominates in it.

It is noteworthy that for three years past the seasons of each year have not kept their ordinary qualities, since the summer has had little warmth and the winter little or no coldness. Also, in all the seasons, continual humidities have exceeded measure with an austral wind, of the nature declared above, and this throughout all of France. I know no man so little versed in natural philosophy or in astrology who does not seek in the air the efficient cause of so many ills which in the space of the said three years have occurred in the kingdom of France. For whence would proceed so many contagious plagues indifferently befallen the old, the young, the poor, and the rich, and in so many diverse places, if not from the air which has not been miserly of its poison but has infected us with it at its pleasure? Whence would have come so many severe coughs,

12

pleurisies, abscesses, catarrhs, discharges, smallpoxes, and galls; so many venomous beasts, as frog, toads, grasshoppers, caterpillars, spiders, flies, locusts, snails, serpents, vipers, adders, lizards, scorpions, and asps, if not from a too great putrefaction which the excessive humidity of the air accompanied by a languid warmth has engendered in us as well as in the universal land of our province? This is how our natural warmth has been enfeebled, how our blood and our humors have been corrupted by the malignity of the air that the austral wind has caused by its hot humidity.

Because of this, this year very little blood has been drawn from any person who has had need of bleeding, whether young or old, wounded or not wounded, of good temperature or of bad, which has not been vitiated and seen to be of white or greenish color. This I have always observed in these last wars and in other places where I was called to cure the wounded or to phlebotomize those who, for precaution as well as for cure of some malady, had blood drawn from themselves by the order of the physicians, in all of whom indifferently I found the blood putrefied and corrupted. This being so, it is a thing more than true that the fleshiness of our bodies can only have been badly disposed, and all our bodies cacochymic since their nourishment, which is the blood, was putrefied and the air wholly corrupted. Thus it follows that the bodies wounded in their fleshy substance were difficult to cure, considering that there was in them destruction of substance, which having need of regeneration of flesh could not bring it to pass whether by medicaments or by artifice of surgeon, so great was its cacochymia. Just as in a hydropic the flesh cannot repair itself because his blood is too cold and aqueous, and as in an elephantiac the flesh and the other parts of the body remain in their putrefaction because of the corrupted blood by which they are nourished, similarly in wounds of cacochymic bodies new acquisition cannot be made nor regeneration of good substance, because in order to return a laudable flesh to the wounded part it is necessary for the blood not to fail in quantity or in quality, especially that the injured part be in its natural temperature. All which things failing in the time of the last wars, it is not astonishing if the wounds, however small and of little consequence, even in the non-noble and principal parts, have brought with themselves so many troublesome complications and finally death, considering that the air which surrounds us, by its inspiration and transpiration, renders wounds putrid and stinking when it is altered and putrid, which the humors prepared for this misfortune also do by their cacochymia.

We have become wise in this by the experience of so many wounds which developed a sea of putrefaction and infection when I was trying to cure them, assuring you that there came from them such a stench that the assistants could smell it only with loathing and with very great difficulty. It must not be alleged that this was for lack of keeping them clean, of dressing them often, nor of administering to them all the necessary things, for such putrefaction was common to princes, to great lords, and to poor soldiers, in whose wounds (if perchance one let a day pass without dressing them, so great was the multitude) one found the next day a great quantity of worms with a marvelous stench. What is more, there occurred to all of them many abscesses in diverse places of their bodies in the parts opposite their wounds. If they were wounded in the right shoulder, the abscess was made in the left knee; and if the wound was in the right leg, the abscess was made in the left arm, as it happened to the late King of Navarre, to Monsieur de Nevers, and to Monsieur de Randan, and to almost all the others. Thus nature seemed so charged with vicious humors that it was not content to purge itself by their wounds alone but sent a portion of its vice into another apparent or concealed place, for if the abscesses did not manifest themselves on the outside, one found them in the internal parts, as in the liver, the lungs, or in the spleen. From the same putrefactions arose some vapors which by their communication with the heart caused continued fevers; with the liver they prevented the pure generation of the blood and with the brain caused alienation of the mind, revery, convulsion, and consequently death. Because of these complications, it has not been possible for any surgeon (however expert he might be) to overcome the malignity of the wounds. For this, however, those who have employed themselves therein are not to be blamed, because it is not possible to fight against God, or against the air, in which often times are hidden the rods of His divine justice.

If, then, following the opinion of the ancient and divine Hippocrates, who says every contused wound must be led to suppuration in order to be cured perfectly, we have striven to do this, and yet we have not succeeded because of the putrefactions, gangrenes, and mortifications which have been put in them by means of the vitiated air, who is it who will justly accuse us for it? Consider also that necessity has forced us to change our fashion of doing and, in place of suppurative medicaments, to use other remedies in order to combat entirely the complications which happened, not only in blows of arquebuses but also swords and other hand sticks, which new remedies can be seen in the reading of this present treatise.

Beyond human causes, the man is badly instructed in the knowledge of celestial things who does not hold for quite certain that the wrath of God looses itself on us to punish the faults that ordinarily we commit against His majesty. His flails have been ready, His rods and His arms have had their ministers always prepared to execute the commandments of His divine justice, in the secrets of which not being able to enter further, I prefer to contain myself in a simplicity than to pass to excess, and to conclude with the best advised that the principal occasion of deaths proceeds from the pure and simple will of God who, by the temperature that His good pleasure has given to the air and to the winds, heralds of His divine justice, has rendered us apt to receive the mishaps which we have incurred by our iniquity.

END

To those who content with healing,
Do not wish to suffer any ill.

AMONG the infinity of so many live reasons,
Among so many arguments, so many naïve lessons,
Which prove, which argue, and which publicly
Show the nature of man obliquely
Incline itself more to evil than good, or to following
The path of virtue, which alone makes us live,
There is none found to my fancy more urgent,
And which contains in itself proof more sufficient,
Than mutual accord, making us avow
The proposal of Epicurus, and to loudly praise the good.
This milk-sop intoxicated with the love of himself
Put the sovereign good in an extreme pleasure,
And for evil exceeding the greatest ills of the world,
Left us pain second to no other.
Since, his soft school allured to the baits
Of a feigned voluptousness, has with so light a step
Run over our universe, that the fool and the sage
Believe all pain to be an extreme rage,
Indeed turn pale in the face, and lose heart,
When they hear pronounced the sole word of pain.
From that have proceeded a thousand lubricous endeavors,
A thousand joyous conversations, a thousand tasteless practices,
Proper for exempting this soft and tender body
From that which indeed can teach him any pain.
But if by his ill luck, he fall in this misfortune
That in some part of him occurs a tumor,
A wound, an ulcer, and that in order to cure him
It is necessary to run to the well-renowned surgeon,
He wishes in the first place that closely he see
To cherishing this body daintily; in order that by carelessness
He suffer no ill, pain, or passion.

If the case requires that one make an incision
Of his already rotted flesh, or that one make opening
By cautery and fires, if the delicate one endure
Any shadow of pain, when its fire has passed,
Oh God! how the troop is eloquent and learned
In speaking ill of that one who following the knowledge
Of the divine Hippocrates has done his duty well.
The one calls him hangman, cruel, inexorable,
The damnable executioner of thousands of bodies;
The other names him donkey driver, who for knowing nothing
Has however amassed an unbelievable wealth.
    There is how our art, which can not healthily
Be exercised by us without giving any
Sentiment of its work, is put in calumny
By those too much devoted to the ease of their life.
    The children of Aesculapius, to whom heaven has disclosed
More secrets in this art than to the remainder
Of all those who were before and after them,
Never knew how to cure a painful member
Without making the patient feel some pain
Which could protect him from his first ill.
Thus by Machaon the foot of Philoctetes
Was finally cleaned, not by a secret
Manner of charming, or by spells or by charms,
Rather by surgery, and by its proper arms;
I mean by its tools and its medicaments,
Which are of this knowledge the proper instruments.
    If then accommodating myself to the fashion of doing
Of the favorites of heaven, I try to please them,
If fleeing imposture and sorcery,
Avoiding abuses, and the buffoonery
Of so many tricksters, I use in all equity
The knowledge that it has pleased the Divinity
To allot to me, as It has seen fit,
Causing sometimes to the ones a notable pain,
To others little or none, according as the greatness
And quality of the ill demands of my labor.
Ought one for recompense insult my effort,
And declare falsely that it is too rude and too sudden?
    I am not a god, who by the sole virtue
Of a word can call forth from the throat

Of a whitened tomb bodies wounded to death,
Nor those which are already delivered to the earth.
I cure by means, which quite as much glory
Merits in its place as other art of which the memory
Has lasted until now, because having taken it
From those who in this case have been better taught,
I have rendered it yet more useful by half,
Easier by a great deal, surer and easier,
By a fine Magazine, in which are contained
More than three hundred tools, of which some are due
To my invention, the rest in the shop
Of my old predecessors have taken their origin.
    As to what of those the greatest part is shown
Portrayed in variable and different display,
Know, friend, that in that I have wished to work
In order more carefully to keep vigil over your health.
Knowing well that the tool made in diverse sorts
Excites in the patient pains more or less strong,
According as it is applied this way or that.
    Thus is the design of my art explained to you
Which never aimed except at relieving the pain
Of the poor afflicted by inhuman pain;
And likewise never wished to flatter
Those whom it behooved to touch to the quick.
For the surgeon with piteous face
Renders the wound of his patient verminous.

The First Book

*treats of wounds made by arquebuses or other firearms
and contains twelve chapters.*

On the Wounds Made

*by arquebuses, or other firearms
and of the complications of these. Book I.*

*Division of the wounds according to the
diversity of the parts injured as well as of the
balls by which they are made. Chapter 1.*

All the wounds that firearms cause in the body of man, simple as well as complicated, with contusion, laceration, irregular temperature, and swelling, are made some in the noble parts, others in the ignoble; some in the fleshy parts, others in the nervous and bony parts; sometimes with rupture and laceration of the great vessels, as of the veins and of the arteries, and sometimes without the rupture of these. Such wounds also are often superficial and often deep enough to penetrate beyond the body and the member in which one receives them. Another diversity is recognized in them according to the difference of the balls, among which are found large ones, medium, and small, as small shot, of which the material (which is ordinarily only of lead) is sometimes changed into steel, iron, or tin, rarely into silver, and even less into gold. Following these variations, the good surgeon is to take different indications for operating and, according to these, to diversify the remedies.

Now, we are not to judge the serious complications of these wounds to arise from the great heat of the ball nor from the poison or other bad quality of the cannon powder, for the reasons that we have treated in the preceding discourse, but because of the contusion, laceration, and fracture that the ball makes in the nervous and bony parts. For when it happens that the ball touches only the fleshy parts and in a body of good temperament, I have formerly found such wounds as little rebellious to cure and as easy to treat as those which are made by other weapons which make round, contused wounds and of such figure as the bullet makes. For this reason, it is necessary to have more consideration for the symptoms or complications of the contusion, laceration, or fracture of bone and violence of the surrounding air than for the heat that one would consider to occur from the bullet and poison of the cannon powder, for the aforesaid reasons. Setting this forth to aid the young and new practitioners in surgery, I have wished to treat it briefly, yet according to what I have been able to experiment in following the wars and what I have continued for the space of thirty years. In this I protest that I have followed the counsel of the physicians and men of my profession most renowned and approved as much for their learning as for long experience. I assure myself that they know things much greater than my writings could contain. Even so, I am not writing for them but for the new apprentices of this art and for those who will have no better aid for relieving the urgent situations arising in such wounds, which surprise sometimes the counsel of the surgeon if reason and experience do not guide his work.

On the signs of the wounds made by arquebuses. Chapter 2.

At the beginning of the treatment, it is necessary to recognize if the wound is made by the blow of an arquebus, which will be easy to see if the figure of the wound is round and livid in color. Similarly, if at the instant that the patient has received the blow he says he felt an aggravating pain as if he had been struck by a great blow with a stone, or that a beam or some other great weight had fallen on the wounded part. Likewise, this is true if little blood issues and the patient feels in it great warmth because of the force of the violent movement and of the strong rush of the air with rupture of the flesh and of the nervous parts. It can be recognized sometimes also by the fractured bones which pierce and press the parts, whence follows discharge and inflammation, and also by the great contusion that the ball makes which cannot enter any part of our body except by great force because of its round figure, as a result of which the place is rendered black by it and the neighboring parts livid. For this reason follow many important complications, as pain, discharge, inflammation, abscess, spasm, delirium, paralysis, gangrene, mortification, and afterward, death.

The means of tending the said wounds at the first dressing. Chapter 3.

For these causes, it is necessary that the surgeon remove properly the foreign bodies, if there are any, such as portions of clothing, wadding, cloth, paper, pieces of harness, links of mail, balls, small shot, bone splinters, lacerated flesh, and other things which can be found in them, and at the first dressing if it is possible, for the complications of pain and sensitivity are not as great at the beginning as in the other times of the malady. Now, to extract them better, it is necessary to put the patient in the position in which he was when he was wounded, because the muscles and other parts otherwise situated can stop and hinder the way. And in order to find the balls and other foreign bodies, it is necessary to search for them with the finger, if it is possible, rather than with another instrument, because the sense of feeling is more certain than any sound or other unfeeling instrument. However, if the ball has sunk quite deeply, then it behooves to search with a sound, round in its extremity for fear of causing pain.

Yet it often happens that by the sound one cannot find the ball, as it befell in the camp of Perpignan to my lord the Marshal de Brissac. He was wounded by an arquebus shot near the right shoulder blade, where several surgeons, not being able to find the ball, said that it had entered into the body, seeing that there appeared no issue. But not having this opinion, I came to search for the ball, and since I did not in any way wish to put the sound to it, I had him make such a gesture of the body as he was doing when he was wounded. Then I gently compressed the parts neighboring the wound. Doing this, I found a swelling and hardness in the flesh with feeling of pain and lividity in the place where the ball was, which was between the lower part of the shoulder blade and about the seventh or eighth vertebra of the back, in which place an incision was made to draw out the ball, by which he was afterward quickly cured. Therefore, it is very good to search for the ball, not only with the sound, but, as I have said above, with the fingers, by handling and treating the place and its surroundings where one conjectures the ball to have been able to penetrate.

Description of the instruments proper for drawing out balls and other foreign bodies. Chapter 4

As for the foreign bodies, they can be drawn out by the instruments hereafter depicted, which are of different shape and size according to necessity. Some are dentelated, others not.

The surgeon must have some of many and different types, some larger, others smaller, in each of these forms, in order to accommodate them to the bodies and to the wounds, and not the bodies or the wounds to these instruments.

INSTRUMENTS REQUIRED TO DRAW OUT FOREIGN BODIES

Dentelated Crow's Beak

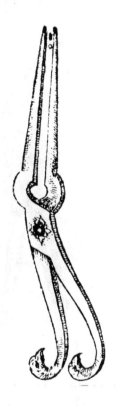

The following is named crane's beak, for the resemblance. This also is dentelated and is proper for extracting from the depth small shot, links of mail, splinters of fractured bones, and other things.

Bent Crane's Beak

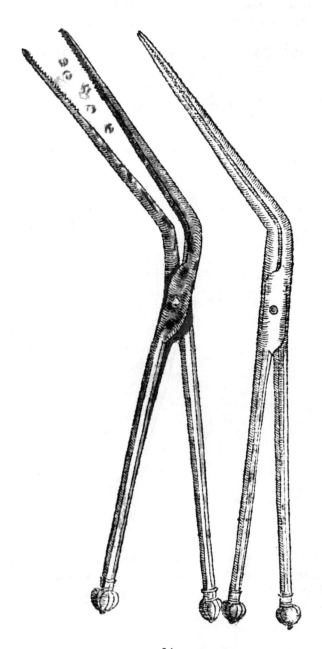

24

Straight Crane's Beak   *Duck's Beak*

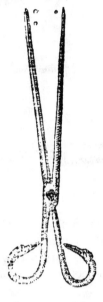 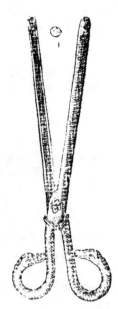

This one, which is named duck's beak, having a cavity in its extremity, broad and round, dentelated in order to take the ball better, is proper principally when the ball is in the fleshy parts.

Another type of ball extractor.

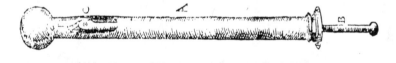

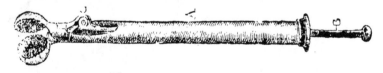

A. Shows its cannula.
B. The rod which makes the hinge open and close.
C. The hinge.

Another figure of ball extractor, named lizard's beak, for drawing out the ball when it is flattened, marked by the same letters as the other.

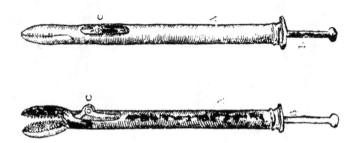

Griffon's Foot

Another type of ball extractor, named griffon's foot, which opens by pulling the rod toward oneself and is closed by passing it inside as is shown to you manifestly, and it is very useful for drawing out balls of cranked arquebuses or others of gross caliber.

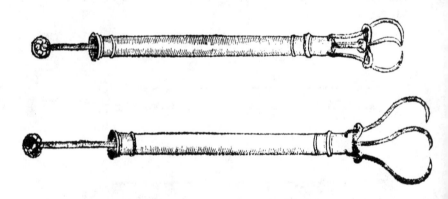

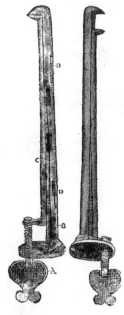

Another instrument, named parrot's beak, for drawing out pieces of harness inserted in the depth of the extremities, even within the bones.

A. Shows the tail of the screw.

B. The barrel.

DD. The chase.

C. The slide, which by means of a screw is raised and lowered.

Another instrument, named swan's beak, which opens with a screw, accompanied by a pincer which heretofore we have named straight crane's beak, and serves to draw out any foreign body after having dilated the wound with the swan's beak.

Swan's Beak

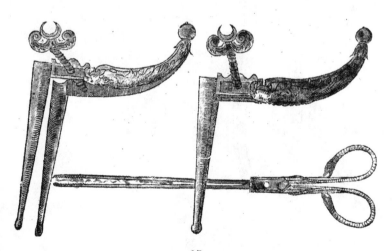

27

Another similar one which opens with a simple hinge.

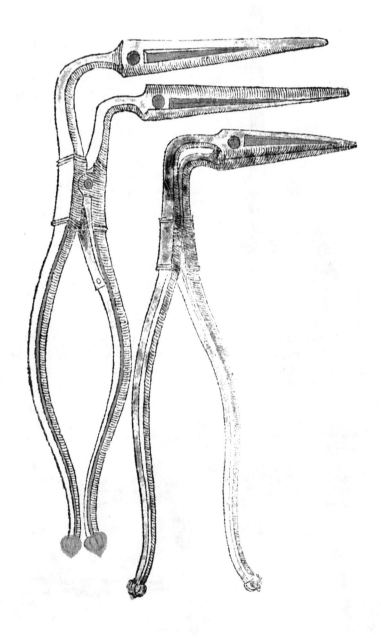

If the foreign bodies, especially the balls and small shots, are superficial, one will be able to draw them out with these, named elevators, which are dentelated inside their extremities in order to do their job better.

Elevators

Another Elevator

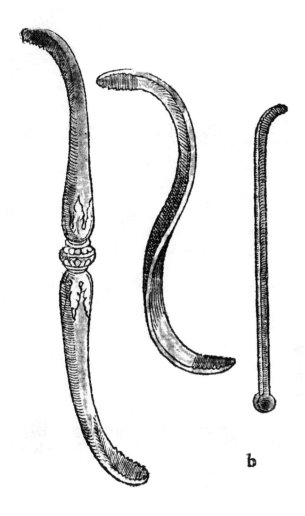

b

Another instrument, named terebra, which turns with a screw within a cannula and is very suitable for drawing out balls when they have penetrated within the bones. For its point enters inside the ball, provided it is of lead or tin (for it could not enter a harder body), and by this means it can be easily taken out.

Terebra

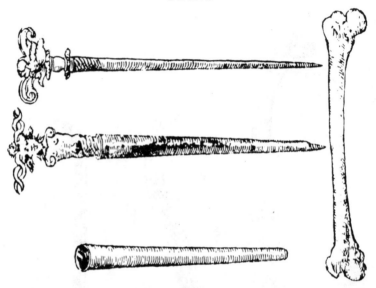

Another terebra, which one uses when the ball is superficial, and not profound.

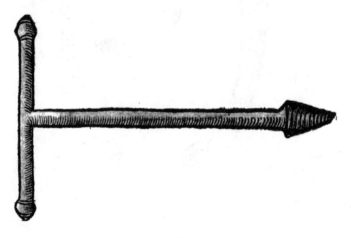

Another terebra; the extremities serve also as elevators.

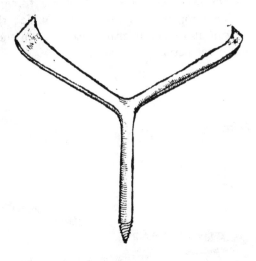

The following is named incisive tenaculum, which is convenient for cutting any fractured bone which appears and is apparent outside the flesh when it has been broken or split by the violence of the blow. And it is easier than a saw is because it does not cause as much pain or stunning; furthermore, its operation is much more sudden.

Incisive Tenaculum

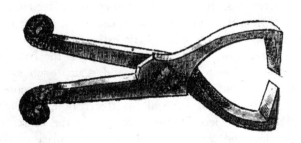

This other is named dilator, which one can use to open and dilate the wounds in order better to find the foreign bodies, for by compressing together two of its extremities, the others are opened. It can also serve in many places, as in the nostrils, in the seat, and other parts.

Dilator

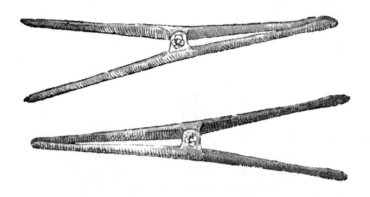

The manner of treating wounds at the first dressing after the foreign bodies are drawn out. Chapter 5.

The instruments which follow are named seton needles, which are suitable when one wishes to pass a seton to hold the wound and the track of the ball open until one has drawn out the foreign bodies which can still be in it. Besides this, they can serve to sound deep wounds in order to find the ball and do not cause any pain because they are round and polished at their extremities. It is necessary then to understand that the sounds with which one searches for the ball are to be moderately large, polished, and round at their extremities, because the walls of the wound and the path through which the ball has passed straightway draw together again and again touch against each other, so that the wound or track appears to the sense of sight much smaller than it is. And for this reason, the slender and sharp sounds are less fit, for they stop in the nearer and contiguous flesh and cannot as easily go to the place of the ball as those that are moderately large. Furthermore, they prick the flesh of the wound and doing this molest the patient very much. This is often the reason that the balls cannot be found. One is also to have larger ones in order to pass through a thigh when the case requires it. Even so, the length of these is to change according to the thickness of the wounded member.

Sounds which are to be of the length of a foot.

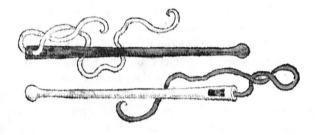

After having drawn out the foreign bodies by the above means, the principal intention will be to battle against the alteration of the air, against the putrefaction of the wound and the complications, which will be done by remedies taken internally as well as by others applied outside and also put within the wounds. Those which are to be administered internally will be taken by the counsel and prescription of the prudent physician, to whose doctrine I leave all that can appertain to the manner of living and to the purgation of the patient. Then the surgeon in his first dressing will apply to the wounds remedies opposing the putrefaction, as is the ointment which follows:

℞ of powder of rock alum, of verdigris, of Roman vitriol, of rose honey, of each ℥ ii, of good vinegar as much as suffices. Let all be boiled together according to the art and let medicine be made in the form of honey.

The virtues of this ointment are that by its warmth and thinness it cuts and attenuates the humors, returns the natural warmth which has been repulsed by the strong impulse of the blow and violent agitation of the air caused by the ball. Further, it corrects the putrefaction of the virulent humor which promptly moistens the crushed and bruised flesh so strongly that it makes a scab. This ointment every and as many times as there will be need of it, can be applied with tents or setons, being dissolved with wine or brandy or, in order to flow better to the depth of the wounds, can be injected with a syringe. What is more, its virtue and strength will be diminished according to the temperament of the bodies and sensitivity of the wounded parts. When the wound is in the nervous parts, it should be mixed with oils of turpentine and of hypericum in such quantity as the expert surgeon will recognize to be necessary. Such an Egyptiac one can and ought to get along without, using none of it at all when we do not have to combat pestilent and pernicious weather for such wounds, such as has been seen the past years. After the use of the Egyptiac, one will make the scab fall and separate with emollient and mild things such as the oil which follows, making it more than tepidly warm.

℞ of violet oil lbs. iiii. In which let two newly born puppies be cooked until the bones dissolve, adding of earthworms prepared as is fitting, lb. i. Let them be cooked together on a slow fire, then let expression be made which will serve for the use aforesaid.

The oil is of great and marvelous efficacy for appeasing the pain as well as for suppurating the wound and making the scab fall. If this one is not available it is necessary to apply that which follows, which is easier to find:

℞ of oil of flaxseed and of lilies, of each ℥ iii, of basilicon ointment ℥ i. Let them be liquefied together, and with these let as much as suffices be applied to the wound.

I well know that the said oils, applied moderately warm, soothe the pain, lubricate, relax, and moisten the walls of the wound, leading it to suppuration, which is the true manner of curing such wounds. Galen quotes Hippocrates, saying, if the flesh is contused, bruised, or beaten by some dart or in other manner, that it must be medicated in such a way that it suppurates the soonest possible. For by this means it will be less molested by phlegmon. Also, it is necessary for the contused and beaten flesh to be putrefied, liquefied, and converted into pus, then afterward new flesh formed. This done, to the parts above and surrounding the wound, it is necessary to apply cooling and strengthening remedies to push back and prevent the discharge of the humors, as this one:

℞ of powder of Armenian bole, of dragon's blood, of powder of myrtle, of each ℥ i, of juice of nightshade, of leek, of purslane, of each ℥ i ss, albumen of iiii eggs, of oxirrhodin as much as suffices. Let liniment be made as is fitting, and others similar, which it is well to use until one is assured of the complications. Similarly, it is necessary not to fail to bandage the member well, placing it in medium position without pain, if it is possible.

How the said wounds must be treated after the first dressing. Chapter 6.

In the second dressing and others following, it is necessary to use only one of the said oils, adding to it some yolks of eggs with a little saffron. One will continue this until the discharge from the wound is digested and turned to suppuration. In such a wound one is to note well that the pus is a longer time in being made than in other wounds made by other instruments because the ball and the air that it pushes before itself dissipates (because of its great contusion) the natural warmth and the spirits of the part. As a result, the tissue breakdown is not so soon or so well made in default of the natural warmth, and there occurs a very great stinking in the discharge and other very dangerous complications.

These things done, there will be need of cleansing the wound little by little by adding to the above medicament turpentine washed in water of roses or of barley or the like, in order to diminish its warmth and sharpness. If the disposition of the weather were very cold, one could add brandy to it, following the counsel of Galen* who teaches that in winter it is necessary to apply warmer medicaments, and in summer less. Afterward we must use this cleanser:

℞ of water of decoction of barley as much as suffices, of juice of plantain, of celery, of agrimony, of lesser centaury, of each ℥ i. Let all be boiled together; at the end of the decoction add Venice turpentine ℥ iii, of rose honey ℥ ii, of flour of barley ℥ iii, of crocus ℈ i, let all be mixed together stirring well; let cleanser be made of medium consistency.

Another:

℞ of juice of climeni, of plantain, of absinthe, of celery, of each ℥ ii, of Venice turpentine ℥ iiii, of syrup of absinthe and of rose honey, of each ℥ ii. Let all boil according to the art, then let them be strained and in the straining add powder of aloes, of mastic, of Florentine iris, of flour of barley, of each ℥ i. Let cleanser be made for the use said.

Or this one:

℞ of Venice turpentine washed in rose water ℥ v, of rose oil ℥ i, of rose honey ℥ iii, of myrrh, of aloes, of mastic, of round birthwort, of each ℥ i ss, of flour of barley ℥ iii. Mix, let

---

*Of the Method

cleanser be made which will be applied within the wound with tents or setons neither too long nor too thick, because they could prevent the evacuation of the discharge and the vapors raised by the wounds, in which, if the vapors are retained, it is a sure thing that they become heated and acquire an acrimony which afterwards erodes the walls and sides of the wound, whence ensue pain, discharge, inflammation, flow of blood, abscess and putrefaction which are communicated to the noble parts, and thereafter cause many pernicious complications. Therefore, the surgeon must not doubt at all that such wounds can adhere and close, because flesh so greatly contused and lacerated cannot be consolidated unless the contusion and the bruise be first suppurated and cleansed. Because of this, I counsel him not to use setons and tents if they are not small and slender so that they do not prevent the issue of the matters and that the patient may suffer them easily, in order to avoid the aforesaid complications. The use of tents and setons is in order to carry the remedies to the depth of the wounds and to hold them open, principally in the orifice, until the foreign bodies have been extracted. And if the wound is sinusal and deep so that the medicaments cannot reach all the injured parts, then it will be necessary to inject the decoction which follows:

℞ of barley water lb. iiii, of agrimony, of lesser centaury, of Alexandrian laurel, of absinthe, of plantain, of each m. ss, of root of round birthwort ℥ ss. Let decoction be made to lb. i, in the expressed straining dissolve of hepatic aloes ℥ iii, of rose honey ℥ ii, let them boil a little.

Then let injection be made within the wound three or four times at each hour that the patient is dressed. And if this remedy is not sufficient to clean the discharge and consume the dead or putrefied spongy flesh, it is necessary to add in the decoction liquified Egyptiac in such quantity as necessity will command, as for one pound of the said decoction about one ounce of the said Egyptiac more or less, which is of very great efficacy for correcting the spongy and bad flesh in the depth of the said wounds. This is done also by the said Egyptiac's being applied alone on the growth of the bad flesh. I have likewise used the powder of mercury and burnt alum mixed in equal portions and found in such case a value quite parallel to that of sublimate or of arsenic (although it is not as painful) and that it makes a very great scab, at which I have often marveled. Some practitioners most often leave a great quantity of decoction in the depth of sinusal wounds, which I do not approve, for it holds the parts extended (which is an abnormal thing to them) and moistens them, which causes nature not to be able to do her duty in regenerating the flesh. Considering that for the cure of any ulcer, as far as it is ulcer, as Hippocrates says, the goal ought to tend to drying and not to moistening. Many err also in the too frequent and assiduous use of setons, in that not adjusting themselves to reason, they keep on renewing them and make them rub the walls of the wounds, by which rubbing they cause pain to the said wounds and cause in them other bad complications. However, I prefer tents more where there is room for them, while, with a great quantity of discharge, cannulae made of gold, silver, or of lead, as are these:

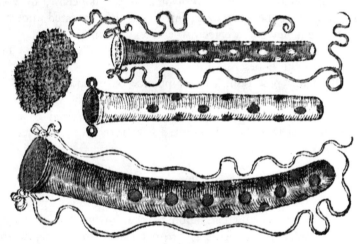

Also, it is necessary to apply compresses on the site of the bottom of the sinus in order to compress the parts distant from the orifice and drive away the discharge. It is especially fitting for the compress to be pierced at the place of the orifice of the sinusal ulcer and above the cannulated tents, and that a sponge be put in it such as you see in this figure, to receive the discharge or pus. By this means expulsion, evacuation and consumption of the discharge will be made much better by beginning the binding at the bottom of the sinus and compressing it moderately so that the matter is not retained inside. The bandages and compresses proper for this operation will be moistened in oxycrate, in sour wine, or in some other astringent liquid to strengthen the part and prevent the discharge, but care must be taken not to constrict the part too much, because by that constriction a pain would be caused by the prevention of the exhalation of the noxious vaporous elements. Likewise, some atrophy could be included in the member.

On the means of drawing out the foreign bodies which have been retained. Chapter 7.

And where there have been some bone splinters which at the beginning were not removed by the aforesaid instruments, then it will be necessary to apply this remedy, having great power to attract them and other foreign bodies:

℞ of roots of Florentine iris, of all-heal and of capers of each ℥ ii, of round birthwort, of manna, of frankincense, of each ℥ i. Let them be pulverized finely and incorporated together with rose honey and Venice turpentine, of each ℥ ii.

Another remedy for removing the said splinters and corruption from the bones:

℞ of dry pine resin ℥ iii, of pumice burnt and quenched in white wine, of iris, of birthwort, of each ℥ ss. of frankincense ℥ i, of scales of copper ℥ ii. Let all be pulverized together diligently, let them be incorporated with rose honey, let cleanser be made.

On the indications which must be observed in the wounds. Chapter 8.

The cleansing and extraction of the foreign bodies having been completed it is necessary to aid nature to regenerate the flesh and to cicatrize. Then, to apply the medicaments suitable to this, it is necessary to proceed by certain indications which are taken, first from the essence of the malady and from the cause of it, if it is present. Although from the original cause (according to Galen in the third book of the *Method*) is not to be taken indication any more than from the weather, which he conceives of as an unapparent cause, and from the past weather. Similarly, it is necessary to take indication from the entire course of the curable malady, that is from the beginning, increase, state, and decline, according to which it is necessary to diversify the remedies.

Another indication is taken from the temperament of the

patient, which also changes the treatment. Every rational and methodical surgeon understands well that other remedies are necessary to a choleric than to a phlegmatic, and thus of the other temperaments, simple as well as compound. Under this indication of temperament is comprised that of age, which does not receive all remedies indifferently but requires some for young persons and others for the old. Further, indication is to be taken from the patient's custom of living. If he had been accustomed to eating and drinking a great deal, and at all hours, then it will not be necessary to prescribe for him as careful a diet as for the one who is accustomed to eat and drink little, and at certain hours. Therefore, diets of panadas are not as proper to the French as to the Italians because it is necessary to relax and restore something to the custom which is of another type. Under this accustomed manner of living can be understood the condition of life and the exercise of the patient, according to his estate. It is necessary to use stronger remedies in the case of rustics, of laborers, and those who have hard flesh, than is necessary in the case of the delicate who work little and do little exercise. Although some have preferred to include this indication under the temperament, for my part I shall not dispute of it, leaving the more complete resolution to the doctors. The indication based on the strength of the patient is to be respected above all others because this failing or being very weak, it is absolutely necessary to neglect all other things to relieve it, as when necessity forces us to cut off a member or to make some great incisions or other similar things. When the patient has not sufficient strength to tolerate the pain, it is necessary to defer such operations (if it is possible) until nature is restored and he has recovered his strength by good food and rest.

Another indication can be taken from the air which surrounds us, under which are comprised the season of the year, the region, the place of our dwelling, and the constitution of the weather. For according to the heat, cold, dryness, and humidity and according also to the continuation of these qualities, it is necessary to adapt the remedies. Thus Guidon said that ulcers of the head were more difficult to cure at Paris than in Avignon, and ulcers of the leg more troublesome in Avignon than at Paris, for the reason that at Paris the air is colder and more humid, which is a contrary thing principally to ulcers of the head. On the contrary, in Avignon the warmth of the surrounding air is the cause of liquefying and subtilizing the humors. Thus more easily and in greater abundance the humors flow downward to the legs, whence it comes that the cure of the legs is more difficult in Avignon than at Paris. But if some allege experience to the contrary, and that wounds of the head are more often lethal or deadly in the warm regions, I shall answer that this does not occur by reason of the air, inasmuch as it is warmer and drier, but by reason of some excessive humidity or bad vapor communicated to the air, as in the places of Provence and Italy, neighboring the Mediterranean Sea.

The indication of curing can also be taken from the temperament of the wounded parts, for the fleshy call for different remedies than bones or nervous parts, or others. Along with other things, the sensitivity of the parts changes the treatment. Since this is true, it is not proper to apply medicaments as acrid and violent to the nerves and tendons as to the ligaments and other insensitive parts. The importance and function of the parts give less privilege of producing a cure. For if the wound is in the brain or in any of the vital and natural parts, it is necessary, according to their importance and action, to change and apply the remedies, seeing especially that for the selection of these, one often makes certain of the prognosis of the outcome, because wounds which penetrate to the ventricle of the brain, to the heart, to the great vessels, to the thorax, to the nervous part of the diaphragm, to the liver, to the lumen, to the small intestines, and to the bladder, if they are great, are necessarily mortal. Also those which are in the joints or near these, and in cacochymic bodies are most often mortal. Similarly, it is necessary not to forget the indications taken from the disposition and connection of the affected part, nor even from its position, as Galen has sufficiently explained in the seventh book of his *Method*, and in the second *To Glaucon*.

Further, in taking the said indications, it is necessary to consider if there is a complication of the malady or not. For thus as the simple malady proposes a simple indication, also the complication and disposition contrary to nature propose complicated indications. Now complications occur in three manners, that is malady with malady, as wound with abscess or fracture of bone; malady with cause, as ulcer with discharge; and malady with symptom, as wound with pain or flow of blood; or all things contrary to nature together, as malady, cause, and symptom. Now to know how to treat all these complications skillfully, one is to follow the doctrine of Galen in the seventh book of the *Method* which exhorts us to consider in complicated affections the most urgent, the cause, that without which the malady cannot be removed. These are things of great importance in every cure. And where the empiric physician has default of counsel, the rational is directed by these three little golden words, on which depend the order and method of proceeding in these dispositions. The symptoms, insomuch as they are symptoms, do not give any indication and do not change the order of cure, because in removing the malady which is the cause of the symptom, the symptom is taken away, for the symptom depends on the malady, as the shadow on the body. Often, however, we are constrained to leave the malady in an unusual cure in order to remedy the complications of the malady, which, if they are urgent, take the place of the cause and not properly of the symptoms. For conclusion, all the above indications are only in order to come to two ends, that is, to return the part into its natural temperament and see that the blood does not fail either in quantity or in quality. That done, as Galen says*, nothing will prevent the regeneration of the flesh and the union of the ulcer from being made. But sometimes it is not possible to put the said indications into execution because of the greatness of the wound, or through excess and inobedience of the patient, or by reason of some other dispositions which have occurred by the ignorance of the surgeon, or bad and undue application of medicaments. As a result, by means of these things, occur great pains, fevers, abscesses, gangrenes (commonly and abusively called esthiomenes) and mortifications, and often death.

How the surgeon, being guided by the above indications, will be able to pursue the treatment of the said wounds. Chapter 9.

At the beginning, then, it is quite necessary to pay heed to relieve the pain by repelling the discharges, by ordering regimen on the six non-natural things and their appendants,

---

Method, bk. III

by avoiding heating and acrid things, and by taking away or diminishing the wine, for fear that it may warm, subtilize, and make flow the humors. And it will be only good at the beginning if there is a discharge of blood to let it flow moderately, in order to purge the body and the part. And where it may not have flowed sufficiently, it will be necessary the following day to use phlebotomy as a counter-irritant and to draw some of the blood according to the plethora and strength of the patient. It is necessary also not to fear directing the flow of blood toward the noble parts. For, as we have said, there is no venomous quality in it.

Yet we will note that such wounds infrequently and at the instant scarcely throw out any blood because the great contusion made by the ball and the force of the agitated air are the cause of pushing the spirits back inside and in the parts neighboring the wound, as we have said before. This is ordinarily recognized in those from whom a large bullet has carried away an extremity, for at the hour of their wounding only a very little blood issues from the wound; nevertheless, there are great veins and arteries torn and lacerated. But some time afterward, as on the fourth, fifth, and sixth day, and sometimes later, the blood will flow in great abundance because the natural warmth and spirits return there. As for purgative medicines, I leave them to the honorable doctors. Yet in the absence of these, it is necessary to give laxatives and move the bowels of the patient at least once a day, either by art or by nature.

The pain is to be appeased according to the manner and remission of it, and in order to remedy it, if perchance there is inflammation, one will apply as local medicament nutritive ointment composed with juice of plantain, jubarb, morel, and their like. The diachalcytheos ointment described by Galen in his first book of the *Composition of Medicaments*, and liquefied with oil of poppy, of roses and vinegar, is not of less efficacy, nor the ointment of bole, nor many others of such faculty, although they are not properly anodynes (for all anodynes are warm to the first degree) and the abovesaid medicaments are cold not so much that they are narcotics (which are cold to the fourth degree). But what? The ointments mentioned in the above case appease pain satisfactorily because they oppose fevers and the flow of humors, often acrid and bilious, which flow faster than the cold and cause greater pain. After the use of repellents, I approve marvelously this cataplasm:

℞ of bread crumbs steeped in cow's milk lb. i ss; let them boil a little adding violet oil and rose oil, of each ℥ iii, of yolks of eggs four in number, of powder of red roses, of flowers of camomile and of melilot, of each ℥ ii, of flour of beans and of barley, of each ℥ i. Mix, let cataplasm be made according to the art.

Or, for a remedy easier to come by, you can take bread crumbs which you will boil a little with oxycrate and rose oil. For the cure of abscesses, it is well also to change the medicaments according to the times of these. For some medicaments are proper at the beginning, others at the increase, and others at other times, as is sufficiently declared in the treatment of the abscesses by Guidon and by those who have written of it. And where nature would tend to suppuration, it would behoove to follow her (as Hippocrates says), for the physician and surgeon are only assistants and aids of nature to help her in that to which she aptly tends.

On the balls which remain in some parts a long time after the cure of the wounds. Chapter 10.

Sometimes balls made of lead remain a long time within the members without there occurring any bad complication or hindrance of consolidating the wound. This I have often seen happen after as long a space of time as two or three years or more. The balls were pushed out by expulsive force and descended by their gravity and heaviness into the lower parts, in which they manifested themselves. Then they were drawn out by operation of the surgeon. Such a long stay in the body without any putrefaction or bad complication, according to my belief, proceeds only from the material of the lead, of which the said ball is composed, it being a fact that the lead has a certain familiarity and acquaintance principally with the nature of the fleshy parts, as we see by ordinary experience which teaches us that lead applied on the outside has the virtue of closing and cicatrizing old ulcers. But if the ball were of stone, iron, or other metal, it is a thing quite assured that it could not remain long in the body, because iron rusts and because of this corrodes the part, which brings at the same time pernicious complications. But if the bullet were in nervous parts or in the

43

noble, even though it were of lead, it could scarcely remain there without causing very great mishaps. Wherefore, if it happens that it remains a long time, it will be in the fleshy parts and in bodies which will be of good temperament and habit. Otherwise, it cannot remain there without inducing pain and many other grievous ills, as has been said.

On the great contusions and lacerations made by artillery bullets and other great cannon. Chapter 11.

Moreover, if a great piece of artillery strikes against an extremity, it often carries it away or wholly breaks and crushes it in such a fashion that the bullet by its great force crushes and breaks not only the bones that it touches but also those that are far from them, because the bone, which is hard, makes resistance and by this means the ball forces it further. That this is true, we see ordinarily in the artillery which has greater action against a wall than it does against a gabion filled with earth, or a ball of wool and other soft things, as we have said heretofore.

However, one should not be surprised if in wounds made by arquebuses occur pain, inflammation, fever, spasm, abscess, gangrene, mortification, and most often death. For severe contusions of the nervous parts, fractures, or strong concussions of the bones made by bullets produce grievous complications, not from the combustion or poison of the powder, as many think, not considering the nature of the said powder, which (as I have said) is not poisonous. For if the wound is made in a fleshy part without touching the nervous parts, it requires for its treatment only remedies similar to those which other contused wounds do, except (as I have said above) the putrefaction caused by the surrounding air, which these past years has altered the wounds for us and caused great putrefaction of the flesh as well as of the bones, from which (as I have said) many vapors have risen to the brain, to the heart, and to the liver, whence there have ensued very evil complications and thereafter death.

*On the means that must be held to rectify the air and to
strengthen the noble parts and fortify the whole body.
Chapter 12.*

Therefore the surgeon must pay heed to administering all
the things which have the power of rectifying the ambient air
and of strengthening the noble parts, also of fortifying the
whole body. This will be done by the things which follow,
administered internally as well as externally. The patient will
take internally in the morning three hours before the meal,
tablets of abbot's diarhodon, or of rose aromatic, of selected
sandalwood, diamoscon, Galen's laeticans and others similar. Externally poultices will be applied over the heart and liver,
somewhat tepid, with a piece of scarlet or sponge, felt or very
delicate cloths. This can serve every surgeon as a formulary:

℞ of rose water ℥ iiii, of water of bugloss, of good vinegar, of each ℥ ii, of prepared coriander ꝫ iiii, of cloves,
of rind of lemon, of each ꝫ i, of red sandalwood ꝫ ss, of both
corals ꝫ i, of camphor ℈ i, of crocus ℈ ss, of powder of abbot's diarhodon ꝫ ii, of theriac and of mithridate, of each ℥ ss,
of powder of flowers of camomile, of melilot, of each p. i; mix,
and let epithem be made.

Further, one is to give often to the patient to smell odoriferous and cooling things in order to strengthen the animal
faculty, as that which follows:

℞ of rose water, of good vinegar ℥ iii, of crushed cloves, of
Galen's theriac, of each ꝫ i; let a handkerchief or sponge be
dipped in this liquid and let the patient put it to his nose often.
He will also use some aromatic pomander for the same purpose,
as this one:

℞ of red roses, of violets, of each ꝫ iii, of bays of myrtle
and of juniper, of red sandalwood, of each ꝫ ii ss, of benzoin
ꝫ i, of camphor ℈ ii. Let powder be made. Afterward:

℞ of oil of rose and of nenuphar, of each ℥ ss, of storax, of
calamite ꝫ ii, of water of roses as much as is sufficient. Let
them be liquefied together with white wax, as much as suffices.
Let cerate for binding the abovesaid powders be made with warm
pestle, and let pomander be made.

Another:

℞ of roots of Florentine iris, of marjoram, of aromatic
calamus, of labdanum, of benzoin, of root ciperus, of cloves, of

45

each ʒ ii, of mosch. gra. iiii. Let powder be made, and with gum tragacanth as much as suffices, let pomander be made.

Another:

℞ of pure labdanum ℥ ii, of benzoin ℥ ss, of storax, of cala., ʒ vi, of Florentine iris ℥ ss, of cloves ʒ iii, of marjoram, of red roses, or aromatic calamus, of each ʒ ss. Let all be pulverized, and let them boil with water of roses, as much as suffices, and let them be strained, and let the straining be liquefied with white wax, as much as suffices, of liquid storax ℥ i, let be made in the fashion of cerate, let them be bound together with a pestle, adding of musk ʒ i; let pomander be made.

Similarly, one can apply frontals in order to strengthen the animal faculty and to provoke sleep and mitigate the pain of the head, as this one:

℞ of rose water ℥ ii, of oil of roses and of poppies, of each ℥ i ss, of good vinegar ℥ i, of troches of camphor ℈ iii; let frontal be made.

One is to fold a cloth in five or six folds and steep it in this mixture, somewhat tepid, and renew it when it is dry. And the head must not be bound very tightly for fear of keeping the pulsation of the arteries of the temples from being free. Otherwise one would increase the pain of the head.*

There are many other external remedies by which one can correct the surrounding air, as making a good fire in the patient's room with wood of juniper, of laurel, of vine twig, of rosemary, of iris root, and also by things spread throughout the room, such as water and vinegar. If the patient is rich, damask water is very proper for it, or the one which follows:

℞ of marjoram, of mint, of roots of cyperus, of aromatic calamus, of sage, of lavander, of fennel, of Stoechades thyme, of flowers of camomile, of melilot, of savory, of bays of laurel and of juniper, of each m. iii, of powder of cloves and nutmegs, of each ℥ i, of water of roses and brandy lb. ii, of good odoriferous white wine lb. x. Let all boil in bain-marie for the use said. Further, one can make perfumes to perfume the said room as these Cyprus birdlets:

℞ of willow charcoal ℥ viii, of pure labdanum ℥ ii, of

---

*Hippocrates, *De vulneribus capitis*

olibanum, of lignum and of bays of juniper, of each ℥ i, of xilaloes, of benzoin, of storax, of calamite, of each ℥ ss, of nutmegs, of sandalwood, of dyer's woad, of each ℈ iii, of cloves, of liquid storax, of each ʒ ii, of zedoary, of aromatic calamus, of each ʒ i, of gum tragacanth, dissolved in rose water, as much as suffices, let be made Cyprian birdlets, or suffitus, in whatever form is agreeable.

As for caries and corruption of the bones, we shall speak of them hereafter amply. Therefore, what we have treated of the wounds made by arquebuses will suffice you for the present, and you will ready yourself for the knowledge of those which are made by arrows, crossbow bolts, darts, lances, and other similar instruments into the discourse of which we now propose to enter.

End of the first book.

The Second Book

treats of wounds made by arrows and similar sticks and contains nine chapters.

The Manner of Treating
Wounds Made by Arrows,

crossbow bolts, darts, lances, and other similar instruments.
Book II.

The differences of wounds made by arrows
and of those which are made by arquebuses.
Chapter 1.

Wounds which are made by arrows, crossbow bolts, or
other similar weapons differ in two ways from those which
are made by arquebuses and other firearms, for sometimes they
are found without contusion, which never happens in wounds
made by firearms. Also, often they are poisonous. According to
these two differences, it is necessary to vary the treatment.
Then it is necessary to consider the different kinds of arrows and
darts because this helps a great deal in the knowledge and
treatment of the wounds.

On the difference of arrows and darts. Chapter 2.

Arrows and darts differ in material, in form or figure,
in magnitude, in number, in manner, and in faculty or force.
The difference in material is that some are made of wood and
others of canes or reeds. Some are garnished at their ends
with iron, lead, tin, bronze, horn, glass, or bone, the others not.
The difference in form is such that some are round, others
angular, some sharp, others barbed in the form of an ear of
wheat. Some have the point extending backward, others down,
and some have a point toward both parts, that is, forward
and backward, some on both sides. Some are broad in front
and cutting in the form of a chisel. As for size, some are
three fingers long, and others medium in length. Number makes
them different in that some are simple, having only a single
point. Others are compounded, having two or many. Also in
these, the manner is diverse. For some have the iron inserted
in the shaft, others have the shaft inserted in the iron. Some
have the iron attached and nailed, others not and hold so
little that in pulling them the iron remains. The faculty makes

49

them differ in that some (as has been said) are poisoned, others not. Such are the special and proper differences of arrows and darts, according to which the wounds that they leave vary the treatment. You can see in this figure the above-said differences:

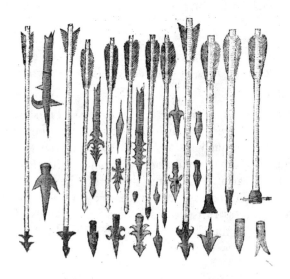

On the difference of the parts wounded. Chapter 3.

These differences revealed, we must next speak of the diversity of the parts affected, which are either fleshy or osseous, some near the joints, others in these; some with great flow of blood and fracture of bone, others not; some are in the principal members, or in members serving these; some deep, others superficial. And if in some of such wounds there appear obvious signs of death, it will be necessary to make a favorable prognosis before touching them, in order not to give an opportunity to the ignorant of speaking ill of our art.

On the extraction of arrows. Chapter 4.

In regard to the extraction of arrows, it is necessary to avoid incising, lacerating, and tearing veins, arteries, nerves, and tendons, if it is possible, for it would be an ignominious thing and against the art if one offended nature more than the arrow did. The manner of drawing them out is double. One is by extraction, and the other by pushing through. However, from the beginning and the first dressing, it is important to remove foreign bodies (if there are any), such as the irons of the arrows, their shaft or wood, and other similar things, as has been said of wounds made by arquebuses, and by the same means. And in order to extract them better, it will be fitting to place the patient in the position that he was in when he was wounded, for the reasons aforesaid, if it is possible, and to use instruments proper to this effect. Of prime use is this one which has a cannula split and dentelated outside, in which is inserted a rod similar to that of the terebra used for an arquebus wound, which has been figured heretofore, except that it is not made with a screw in its extremity. Also, it is larger in order to dilate the cannula to fill the hollow in the iron and extract it from the fleshy parts as well as the osseous, provided that there has not remained any of the wood of the arrow in the hollow of the iron. Another instrument can be used, which is dilated by pressing the two rear extremities, also dentelated outside, as you can see in this figure. The signs for knowing where the iron is are that if one touches the part where it is, one will feel roughness and unevenness. Also, the flesh will appear contused, livid, and black, and the patient will feel heaviness and continual pain in the wounded part.

Instruments proper for extracting the irons of arrows whose shaft is out.

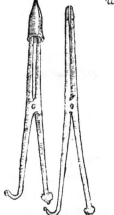
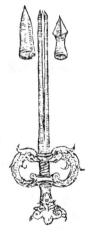

This one is dilated by compressing the grip.

This one opens by a screw which is inserted in its cannula.

Bent crow's beak, proper for drawing out mails and other small foreign bodies, with an instrument closing and opening by a screw, convenient for drawing out the irons of arrows.

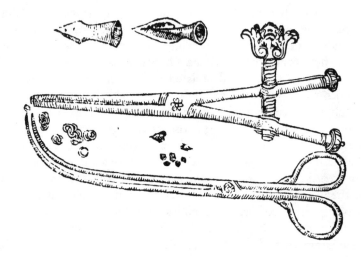

Another small hook for drawing out mails and other foreign bodies which can be hooked, which you can also use for this same effect in wounds from arquebuses.

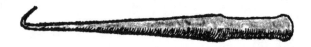

But, if by chance the barbed iron, whether of arrow, pike, dart, or lance, remains in some part of the body as, for example, in the thigh or leg, still with a portion of wood which was broken into splinters, then it will be necessary that the surgeon cut the wood above the splinters with incisive tenacula and then he is to draw out the iron with dentelated tenacula as you can see by this figure:

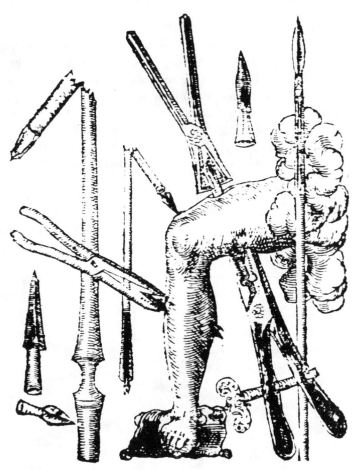

How it is necessary to proceed to extract broken arrows.
Chapter 5.

But if the iron is perchance broken in such a way that one cannot take it with the above tenacula, let it be drawn out (if it is possible) with the crane's beak or crow's beak or other proper instruments, which have been depicted heretofore. And if the shaft is broken so near the iron that one cannot have a hold on the iron nor on the shaft with the crane's beak, then it will be necessary to extract it with the arquebus terebra. For if it inserts itself into lead, with stronger reason it will indeed into wood. Similarly, if the iron were barbed, as the iron of English arrows often is, then if it is possible it is well to push it through the part. For by this means one will avoid greater danger, because in withdrawing it the barbs could break nerves as well as veins, arteries, and other parts. This one is to avoid carefully (as we have already said). Wherefore it is better to make a counteropening on the side opposite the iron and get it out by pushing it through, supposing that there would be there a small thickness to incise. By this means and with less danger the wound can be cleansed and consolidated. On the contrary, if the barbed iron were at the place of a bone or (as often happens) inserted within the depth of the muscles of the thigh, of the arms, of the legs, or of other parts, in which there would be a great distance, then it does not behoove to push it, but rather to dilate the wound, avoiding the nerves and great vessels as does the good and expert anatomical surgeon. Also, it is necessary to apply duly a dilator hollow in its internal part and do this in such a way that one can take the two wings of the iron, then with the crane's beak hold it firm and draw out the three together as this figure below shows us:

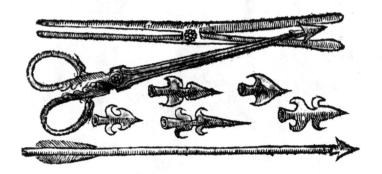

*What must be done if the arrow is inserted
in the bone. Chapter 6.*

Now, if the bolt or arrow is inserted in the bone in a fashion that it cannot be taken out by pushing it through but indeed by drawing it out by the place where it entered, it is well to shake it and move it sagely if perchance it holds strongly. One must take good care that the iron not break, a portion of it remaining in the bone. This you will be able to do by the instrument named crow's beak or others proper for this, figured above. Forthwith, you will not fail to express the blood, letting it flow enough, taking indication of the amount in order that

the part be cleaned and less bothered by inflammation, by putrefaction, and by other evil complications.

How it is necessary to treat wounds made by arrows, after these are extracted. Chapter 7.

The extraction made and the first dressing, if the wound
is simple you will treat it as simple, but if there are complications you will employ yourself according to the complications
of the wound. To appease the pain you will be able to apply
with great profit oil of puppies according to our description
heretofore. And in order to relieve other complications according to the nature and urgency of these, that which is found
in Guidon in the treatise of wounds, and in all the *Method* of
Galen, and especially what we have prescribed in the treatise
of wounds made by arquebuses may be used because they are
almost similar.

On poisoned wounds. Chapter 8.

There remains now to understand and consider that these
wounds are sometimes poisoned (as we have said) and that
that comes from the original cause, arrows thus prepared by the
enemy. This one can recognize as much by the story of the
patient who says he feels great and stinging pain, as if he had
been bitten by wasp flies (principally in warm venoms which are
most often used in such cases), as also by the flesh of the
wounded man, which becomes pale and somewhat livid with
some appearance of gangrene. In such a case, many other more
serious and greater complications happen which do not customarily occur in other wounds where there is no poison. Therefore, from the beginning (after having drawn out the foreign
bodies, if there are any there), it is necessary to make rather
deep scarifications around the wound, applying to it cupping
glasses with considerable flame, in order to attract and evacuate
the virulent matter. Likewise, it is a very useful operation and
of marvelous effect to have the wound sucked by some person
who is not fasting and who first will have washed his mouth
with vinegar in which has been boiled tormentil, Spanish broom,
or white mullein. In default of this remedy one will content
oneself with wine in which some portion of theriac has been
dissolved. The ablution of the mouth made, the sucker will

take some oil in his mouth and will expel it swiftly for fear that the venom may injure it in some way. To obviate which further, it is necessary to take care that he have no ulcer in his mouth and that he wash the wound, before sucking it, with brandy, vinegar, and theriac dissolved together, or other similar things. One can also for this same end use the following remedies:

℞ of wax, of black pitch, of fat of wether, of old oil, of each gill i, of galbanum and of ammoniac, of each ℥ ss, of theriac and of mithridate, of each ℥ ii ss. Let ointment be made as is fitting.

In place of such ointment, such a cataplasm may be made:

℞ two onions, of tips of rue p. ii, of mustard ℨ ii, of common salt ℨ i ss. Let all be crushed with a little fermento and common honey, let cataplasm be made, adding oil of ruthacei ℥ ss.

Another cataplasm which has great force of attracting poison:

℞ of crushed onions ℥ iii, of mustard ℥ i, of common salt ℥ ss, of juice of rue ℥ i, of dove's dung ℥ ss, of garlics cooked under ashes ℥ i ss, of common honey ℥ iiii, of oil of laurel as much as suffices; let cataplasm be made in the form of liquid poultice, and let it be applied rather warm. Plaster for this purpose:

℞ of gum ammoniac, of galbanum, sagapenum, of opopanax, of asafetida ℥ i, of powder of pepper, of live sulphur, of each ℨ vi., of dove's dung ℥ ss, of juices of calamite, of wild mint and wood garlic, of each ℥ i ss; let the gums be dissolved with vinegar and brandy; let plaster be made according to the art.

Another for this purpose:

℞ fermenti acris ℥ ii, of opopanax and of sagapenum dissolved in vinegar and aqua vini, of each ℥ i, of live sulphur ignem non experti, and of common salt, of each ℥ ss, of pulverized round pepper, and of birthwort, of each ℨ ii, of dittany and anagallis, of each ℨ ss, of common honey, of Venice turpentine, of each as much as suffices. Let medicine be made according to the art. It is necessary also to apply vesicatories below the wound. Another cataplasm:

℞ 12 old nuts, as much of garlic, of common salt and of rock salt, of each ℨ i. Let all be incorporated together with honey, let cataplasm be made.

Such medicaments not only have the faculty of attracting and destroying the venom but also hold the lips of the wound wide and open. This it is necessary to do in order that the venomous matter may be discharged, for repellent medication must not be used on the wound before having removed the quality of the venom, especially in the surrounding parts principally when there is some appearance of inflammation; also to prevent the flowing and descent of the humors into the wounded part. Some have recommended, in bites and stings of poisonous beasts, to take fowl and other birds and to pluck their rear and to put inside a grain of salt and to apply it to the wound, then close tightly their beak in order to draw out the venom better. Likewise, they advise obtaining small animals split alive, as dogs, cats, fowl, also lungs of ox, of calf, of sheep, of pig, and others, and to apply them over the lesion as well as over the neighboring parts. This similarly I have found reasonable in venomous wounds made by arrows, because such remedies appease the pain, destroy the poison, and comfort the part. Cauteries, principally the actual, are very convenient for weakening the strength of the venom because they deaden the force and virulence of it and do not permit it to gain further, as will be said at the end of this book. All of these remedies against venom are to be applied straightway and at once (if it is possible) in order that it may not have time to penetrate deeply and to occupy the noble parts, for the remedies would otherwise be useless.

It must not be forgotten to make a ligature above the wound, and that it be rather tight in order that it may hold and can prevent the venom from penetrating and mounting to the internal parts. In compressing the vessels, let it also not be too tight for fear of stupefying and causing to be lost the feeling of the part, which by this means could turn into gangrene. Some say they have made a ligature above bites and stings of poisonous beasts with a branch of Spanish broom or with a stalk of white mullein and affirm that the venom was not able to pass beyond, which I approve. Theriac and mithridate applied alone and put several times in the wound and neighboring parts or dissolved with brandy bring a singular aid, for if one gives the wounded to drink a dram or a half dissolved in white wine or cordial waters, and powder of gentian a dram and a half, the soonest that it can be done, he will feel great alleviation from it. This done, it will be important to obtain suppuration of the wound, the soonest possible, with a digestive composed of yolks of eggs, violet oil, and turpentine of Venice. In all of these medicaments, it must not be omitted to add a little theriac. Having suppurated the wound it is necessary to soften it with such a cleanser:

℞ of Venice turpentine ℥ iiii, of rose honey ℥ i, of rose oil ℥ iii, of powder of root of gentian, of tormentil, of round birthwort, of devil's bite, of each ℈ ii, of brandy a little; let all be incorporated together, let a cleanser be made for the use said.

Moreover, there must be applied on the region of his heart a comforting poultice, of which you will have the description in the treatise on gangrene.

The indication for treatment is to be taken from the alteration of the venom, which causes the pain and other complications, changing and transforming one contrary quantity by another contrary quantity. As an example, if the patient feels a severe coldness in his wound or in his whole body, it is necessary to use warm remedies. On the contrary, if he feels great warmth, one will use cold ones. As for the prescribing of his regimen, any well-experienced surgeon will order it for him according to the six non-natural things always opposing the venom. If it is warm, it is necessary to aim at cooling and if it is cold, to the contrary, for if the venom acts by a specific property, one will overcome it by temperate things, which are of a quality contrary to the said venom.

On the signs of the quality of venoms. Chapter 9.

The signs for recognizing if the venom is warm are great redness, burning, and stinging pain in the part, with swelling and color tending to lividity. The signs of cold venom are numbness or sleepiness, coldness, and soft inflammation in the wounded part. These are often presages of death, when there occurs a cold sweat, a great chilling of the extremities, a spasm and failing of mind, the color changing into greenness, blackness, and lividity. For such signs appearing denote approaching death. Warm poisons are causes of death for the reason that they dissipate natural warmth and inflame the mass of blood by introducing foreign warmth into the heart, and consequently in all the parts of the body, destroying the vital spirits. Cold poisons are causes of death for the reason that they congeal the mass of blood and stupefy the spirits. The others work by occult property, because they are totally contrary to human nature and, applied in as little quantity as one may wish, are still harmful. For this reason, Galen never permits mixing them with the alexipharmics and antidotes for venoms. Actual cauteries applied at the beginning (as has been said) have great efficacy against all venoms because they dissipate, dry, and consume, even blunt and deaden the matter of these venoms. If the said cauteries were of gold, the operation of them would be more exquisite. After their application, it is necessary to aim at the fall of the scab and pursue the treatment, as has been said in the treatise on wounds made by arquebuses.

End of the second book.

On the Fractures of the Bones

Book III.

On the causes and differences of fractures.
Chapter 1.

The causes of fractures are all external things which can crush, break, and shatter the bones in so many fashions that it would be difficult to count the exact number of such causes. However, because fractures occur most often as much by the great violence of the bullets and balls of arquebuses as by these shots, principally from the great crossbow bolts, I have not wished to neglect to write of them according to what I have seen of them by experience. Now, because these fractures are made often lengthwise, at other times across, and sometimes athwart, and also because some are incomplete, others complete, some with even pieces, others dentelated, uneven, and splintery, that is to say, in several pieces, as is a nut broken under a hammer, and then some are made on the surface of the bone with some portion of it like a separate scale, others without the bones being separated from each other, but only split lengthwise. Further, because there are some simple, in which there is neither wound nor other injury, and some compound, which are with other lesions and complications, as wound, flow of blood, contusion, inflammation, gangrene, and similar complications, it is necessary, as I have written heretofore, to consider the part in which the fracture is made, because quite often it occurs to the head, sometimes to the ribs, to the bone of the adjutory, to the bone of the thigh, and to one or to two fociles of the arms as well as of the legs, likewise to the joints and other parts of our body. If the fracture occurs in the joints or near them, then very perilous complications occur, as pains, insomnia, restlessness, fevers, abscesses, delirium, convulsions, and quite often death. Wherefore, according to these differences and indications, it is necessary to vary the treatment and note in this place by manner of warning that Galen in the sixth book of the *Method* says that every solution of continuity made in the bone is named catagma.

On the signs of fractures. Chapter 2.

The signs of fractures are rather evident and manifest, of which the first and the most certain is when in handling the fractured part one finds the parts of the bones separated, and one feels a crepitation and attrition in the bones making noise against each other. Similarly, one recognizes the fracture by the impotence of the part, and especially if the fracture is in the adjutory bones or in the large bone of the leg. For when it is only in the small focile of the arm or of the leg, the patient will in no way leave off using the arm or walking on the foot, because this focile serves only to sustain the muscles and not the body, as does the great focile. Further, the fracture can be recognized by the altered position of the part, accompanied by a very great pain which comes because of the wound of the membrane of the periosteum, of the marrow, and from the compression of the surrounding nervous parts.

On the prognosis of fractures. Chapter 3.

The bones because of their dryness cannot be as easily agglutinated as the flesh is, but around their fracture is formed a hard substance made from what overflows from the nutrition of the broken bone, which substance holds the bone and agglutinates it, with time it hardens so strongly that the place of such agglutination is found firmer and harder than the non-broken part. For as glue serves in wood to join it, similarly the callus serves as the same thing in broken bones to agglutinate and join them together. It is then not without great reason that the fractured bones, to be united together, require great rest. For if one moves the part before the agglutination is perfect, the callus breaks and dissolves. Its material is not to fail in quantity nor in quality any more than the blood in the generation of wasted flesh. And in order to treat it well, it is necessary for the part to be in its natural temperament, otherwise this cannot be done, or at the least it will be retarded. Fractures in the young are much more easily cured than in the old, because the young are still full of glaireous and viscous sap, and abounding in natural, radical and substantific humidity. Although one can allege the elderly have more humidity than the young, which I think I have answered by using this word "substantific and natural humidity," differing from that of the old which is not such, but superfluous and waste material, whence it follows that it is less apt and proper for making the generation of the callus. Fractures made in the adjutory bones and in the large bones of the leg are more difficult to cure than those which are only in one of the fociles, because they are more difficult to hold and because more time is necessary to make the callus. Also, bones which are thin and spongy are more quickly agglutinated by the callus than those which are not of such nature. Moreover, fractured bones in bodies of sanguine temperament are sooner united than in the choleric.

Broken bones are never so well united that there does not remain in them some unevenness and prominence, by reason of the union of the bones made by the callus. Wherefore the surgeon is to make the bandage properly, otherwise the callus will remain larger or smaller than there is need. This is done to hold the bone in its place, also to push back the blood already flowed into the wound and to keep too much of it from coming there. For by a great contusion and fracture of the bone, the blood comes out of the vessels for the reason that they are violently expressed and pressed, which causes an ecchymosis in the flesh, of livid and black color, because the blood outside of its proper vessels has spread out into the flesh and under the skin and in it.

The fracture in which there are sharp and pointed splinters is more difficult and more dangerous than those which have none because the splinters prick the flesh and the other parts, whence follow many dangerous complications. When the bones are not in their natural position, the part falls into atrophy because the veins, arteries, and nerves are perverted from their proper place and because the part does not move at all, or with great difficulty. Wherefore the spirits cannot manifest themselves in it and the nutrition does not come to it in such quantity as is necessary to nourish the part, whence atrophy ensues. This same complication can come through keeping the part bound too long and too tightly.

When the broken member is greatly swollen and inflamed, there is danger in wishing to reduce it that the patient may fall into spasm. Wherefore it is necessary to defer the reduction, if it is possible, until the humors are resolved and the part unswollen. Fractures are united by the callus, some sooner, others later, and it is not possible to give a definite rule for this, as much because of the constitution of the year, of the region, of the temperament of the patient, and of his manner of living, as for the type of the ligature. Also, when the patient is weak, or the humor is aqueous and subtle, then it is not proper for forming the callus. On the contrary, when the forces and virtues are full, then they do their duty in joining the bones together. Even if the matter is gross and thick, it is easily converted into the substance of the callus. Therefore, it is well to prescribe to the patient nourishments and medicaments proper for aiding nature to do this, which we will say hereafter.

On the manner of reducing fractured bones. Chapter 4.

It is necessary for the surgeon, when he wishes to reduce fractured bones, to extend and pull the injured part quite straight. For, the bones being broken, the muscles draw back toward their origin and, therefore, it is impossible to reduce the bones without extending the muscles. The part thus pulled, one will reduce the bones into their place more easily by pressing with the hands the cracked and broken bones which, if they make any prominence, will be compressed and pushed together with bands, compresses, and splints.

On the signs by which one will know the bones
to be well reduced. Chapter 5.

The signs by which one will recognize the reduction to be well made are first taken from the appeased pain, by reason that the fibers of the muscles and other nervous parts are put back in their natural position, and that the bones do not press them any more, and also that in touching one does not feel any prominence, but an evenness. If the fractures are in the thighs and in the legs, in order to know if the bones are well reduced, it is necessary to compare the healthy part with the sick, bringing the feet and knees near each other to see if they are equal in length. This thing one is to observe every time one treats the patient because the fractured bone can move out of its place again by the patient's turning from side to side in his bed or by certain tremors which come when he is sleeping. This is done by the force of the muscles pulling back toward their origin and as a result moving the fractured bone, which by reason of this does not keep the position that the surgeon has given to it but rather rides up on the other, whence the patient feels extreme pain until the bones are again put back in their place. The surgeon is to be very attentive to that, for when the callus forms (if the bones ride up on each other) the bone will remain that much shorter, and, consequently, the member. This will make the patient always limp (to his very great regret, and dishonor of the surgeon). Therefore, it is necessary for the patient to take care of it on his part, keeping himself well from moving the broken part, as much as possible for him, until the callus is stiffened and hardened.

On the manner of treating fractures at the first dressing.
Chapter 6.

Now we shall describe the manner of tying and bandaging the broken bones, which will be practiced according to the form of the fracture occurred, which admonishes us always to lead and guide the bandage toward the side opposite to that to which the fracture is inclined, in order thus to contain the bone in its place. Further, we shall take indication from the part and place in which the fracture is made. For if it is in the arm, one knows well the part of this which is toward the carpus or wrist is not as large as that which is in the middle nor others of the joint of the elbow; similarly, the thigh is not so large near the knee, nor the leg near the ankle bones, as they are higher. Because of this, the good surgeon will fill the small and slender extremities of these parts, in order to make them equal to the larger, with compresses and bandages applied around them in order that the splints and ferules, which can be made of wood, lead, tin, thick cardboard, or the bark of trees, and similarly, the bandages, compress the fractured part evenly. Having reduced the member the nearest that will be possible to its natural figure, it is necessary to apply all around the fracture, especially over it, rose oil with a little vinegar and plasters covered with rose ointment, then to begin the bandage on the fracture and to make three or four turns on it in order to hold the bones better. From there, turn the bandage back upward on the healthy parts, always pulling toward the body, and the farthest from the fracture that one can, until the bandage is all used. By this means, one pushes back the blood which had already flowed to the fracture and in the neighborhood of it. Also, one prevents any more of it from flowing there. Now, if anyone should make the compression otherwise, he would send the blood back to the wounded place and could cause abscesses and other bad complications. For, as Hippocrates says, the blood which flows downward only goes there by one road, but that which is pushed back by the bandage goes by two paths, that is, from high to low, and from low to high, in which case it is necessary to pay heed to drive the great excess of blood toward the body rather than toward the distant parts, because the extremities are not capacious or suitable enough to receive so great an abundance of blood and humors, and especially are not powerful enough to digest them and to assimilate to their substance. What is more, an inflammation and abscess could be formed in them with other perilous complications. But when one pushes it back toward the body, then it is ruled and governed by the natural faculties.

The first bandage completed it is necessary to have a second with which one will likewise commence to bandage on the fracture, but it will make only one turn or two there because it is not necessary to send as great a quantity of blood to the extremities as to the upper parts, for the abovesaid reason. This turn made or these two, it will be guided, tightening it gently, toward the bottom or extremity of the part. Then it will be led back upward, to the place where the first bandage has ended. And its turns or revolutions, or those of another bandage which can be called the third, will be made in the opposite direction. That is, if the first has been led to the right, the second will be guided to the left in order to reduce the muscles into their natural figure and position, which pressed and twisted had changed place according to the revolutions of the first bandage.

The length and width of the bandages cannot well be written, for it is necessary to have them long and wide according to the length and thickness of the fractured members. I do not wish to forget here to warn you, your bandage made, that you must not sew the end of your bandages in the width that they are, for they would not hold so firmly even though they were closely attached, but you must fold them back, lengthwise on one side and the other, making their ends almost in a point. Then you will sew them to fix them. In doing this, you will take care not to make the sewing at the place of the wound, for fear of the pain which would be made in it by attaching them there. It is well also for the bandage and compresses to be steeped and bathed in oxycrate or in thick, sour wine and other similar liquids, quickened on the fire. It will be necessary to moisten them often, especially in summer. By this means, one strengthens the part by pushing back the edema, and consequently one prevents the inflammation and the pain. The member thus bandaged, our art commands to place it in its proper and accustomed position in order that the patient can last long in it. This position will be found laudable and good if the muscles are in their place and as high as possible, but without pain. This will be done if the member is held in medium position. This done, one will be able to ask him if he is not too confined, and if he says no, except a little over the fracture, then it will be necessary to conclude that it is well.

On the complications which come from badly made compression. Chapter 7.

The too-tight compression excites pain, inflammation, gangrene, and mortification*. That which is not tight enough profits nothing to the fracture. On which it must be noted that if on the morrow of the first dressing there occurs in the part a small soft swelling, it is a sign that the compression is well made and that it has driven away and expressed the blood from the fractured part. But if the swelling is large and hard, it is a sign that the compression is too tight, wherefore it behooves to loosen it promptly and to foment it with warm water and with oil, then to tighten it again moderately.

Now, if the patient is without great pain, it is well to leave him three or four days, more or less, without untying him. And when one removes the bandages, if one finds the bandages

---

*Hippocrates, *On Fractures*

very loose because of the destroyed and resolved swelling, it will be a good sign, for by the compression the blood has been expressed from the part, whence it is rendered smaller and slenderer. If there occurs in the part a pruritus or itching, which is made at the beginning because the vapors cannot be freely exhaled because the part is pressed and covered with plasters, compresses, and bands, besides the fact that it remains without its accustomed exercise and therefore there is less natural warmth, then it will behoove to untie the bandages every three days in order to give air and transpiration to the dark excretions and seropurulence contained beneath the skin, for fear that they may break and ulcerate the part, which has happened to many through lack of doing this. Likewise, it is necessary to forment the part with warm water, also to use light frictions with the hand or warm cloths, with which one will rub it in all directions, that is upward, downward, to right, to left, to and fro, across and around, for such friction destroys the superfluous vapors contained in the part. Similarly, one can use fomentations of sage, of camomile, roses, melilot, and the like, boiled in water and wine. But if by chance there occurs a swelling in the hand, the knee, or in the foot because of some broken bone, in consideration of this, it is necessary to begin to bind and tie these parts rather than the fracture. For if one did otherwise, the humor contained in this swelling and which flows to it continually could not be sent back to the upper parts because of the compression that the first pressure dressing would make.

Having thus discoursed on fractures in general, now I shall treat of the particular which occur in the arm and in the legs only. For it is not my intention for the present to pass further beyond, because of the rest I shall speak of them more amply in my general practice.

On the fracture of the adjutory bone, called os brachii.
Chapter 8.

If the extremities of this bone ride up much on each other and if this is a very robust man, then it is well to make great extension to the arm, having made the patient sit rather low in order that he can not rise when one reduces the fracture, and also so that the surgeon may do the operation more at his ease. Now to prevent his getting up, one can bind him in a suitable way, to the end that he hold himself stable. Because this bone is somewhat arched toward the exterior part, there is need to put some folded cloth between this bone and the side for fear that, the reduction made, the fracture may incline too much toward the inside. For the bones which are arched and bossed toward the exterior part are given proper shape when they are pushed in the opposite direction. Similarly, it is necessary not to fail in making the extension to pull the arm downward in a straight line, as though one wished to put it in a scarf. For if one wished to make the reduction with the arm raised and extended or in some other position, it would be necessary to hold it always in the same situation and position in which one would have reduced it. Thus it would come about that the reduction could easily be undone when one wished to hang the arm in a scarf, which is very necessary to be observed in putting back the said broken bone, holding the arm couched almost against the body and hanging toward the waist. In this case, the surgeon will take care bandaging it and putting on it compresses and splints in the fashion above. In such fractures the arm remains impotent and without any movement until the callus is made, which is made in this bone in forty days and sometimes sooner, other times later, for which one cannot give a rule.

On the fracture of the fociles of the arm as well as of the leg. Chapter 9.

But if the fracture is only in one of the two fociles, the arm for that will not remain altogether impotent. Rather, it will be usable because the other will support the default of the one which is fractured. Similarly, if only the little focile of the leg named sura is broken, the patient will still be able to walk. But if it is the large one name tibia, even though the little one is entire, he will remain impotent until the callus is made because this bone sustains the body and not the little one, which is made only to serve as support to the muscles, besides the fact it does not have movement as the large one. Therefore, if both the fociles of the arm are broken the treatment of it is more difficult because they are more difficult to hold than when there is only one of them, for the one which remains entire still sustains the arm and keeps the muscles from drawing back toward their origin as they do when both are broken. Also, to reduce them, greater extension must be made. If the fracture is accompanied by a wound, you will take care to reduce it well and to sustain the arm with bent plates of tin and a small pillow, as you can understand by this figure, and to treat the wound as you will hear hereafter in the fracture of a leg with wound.

The arm is to be situated comfortably and to hang in a scarf so that the hand is scarcely higher than the elbow, in order that the blood and the humors do not fall on the hand, which likewise will be situated and held in a supine position, if it is

The figure of an arm broken with wound.

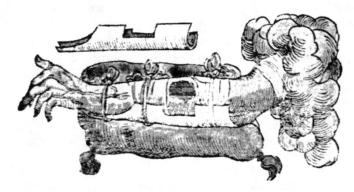

possible, that is, the palm toward the sky or approaching such situation and position, for fear that after the cure, the action of the arm may be marred. For, if the position of the hand is made otherwise than I say and as is practiced ordinarily, that is, the two fociles crossing each other in Burgundian cross and the hand prone, the position remains vitiated when the bones knit again, and consequently the movement marred, as has happened to many who afterward cannot extend the supine hand. Further, you will not forget to flex and at times extend the arm of the patient (however, without violence) in order to prevent the discharge which is made in the joint of the elbow from hindering the bones from being agglutinated together, which is done quite often, whence ensues immobility of the said joint, as if there were a callus formed in it, and hence afterward it comes about that the arm can not be bent or extended, as I have seen happen to many and also Galen has left it to us in writing.*

On the fracture of the bone of the thigh, called os femoris. Chapter 10.

One commonly finds that the extremities of the bone of the thigh, when broken, ride up on each other because of the great and strong muscles which are in it, which then draw back toward their origin, as we have said heretofore. Therefore, when one will reduce the fracture of this bone, it is necessary for the surgeon to pull and extend the thigh very strongly, aided in doing this by strong and powerful men and assistants in order to bring the ends of the broken bones back against each other. And to this end, the ancients had invented this instrument named glossocomium:

Figure of an instrument named glossocomium.

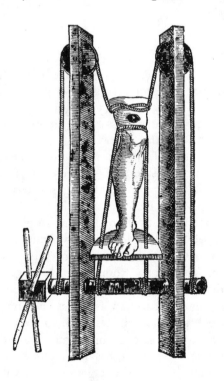

---

*Galen, *In Hippocratis de articulis librum.*

Then also let him consider that this bone is not at all of straight figure, as we have said of the adjutory bone, but arched in front and in the exterior part, for its interior part is concave, as you see manifestly by these figures:

Figure of the thigh bone called os femoris.

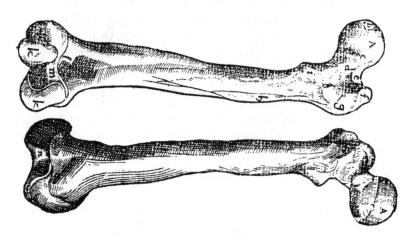

Therefore, if the said os femoris is not well reduced, and if one does not put good compresses and bandages on it, it often turns out to the contrary of good. For this reason, it is necessary to apply a compress to the inside of the thigh which will fill the flat and the concavity of it for fear that the bone may dislocate itself from its place and, knitting again, may change its natural position. Having used this fashion of practicing, one will recognize by the signs heretofore written the reduction of the fractured member to be well made. Therefore, it is necessary for the patient for his part to give good care to it, holding himself stable and quiet without moving the part. Also, it is necessary for the surgeon, as much as he can, to compress the muscles by compresses, bandages, sticks, splints, ferules, and pads of straw. These will be so long that they will be put on from the os ilium as far as the end of the foot, in order to hold the bone better and to keep the patient, in turning from side to side, from putting the reduced bone out of the place into which it has been put back. However, he must guard himself from pressing too much with the said pads and splints the protuberances of the bones, such as the ankle bones of the foot, and protuberances of the knee and others, and likewise the nerves and tendons. According to Hippocrates, one can call the boxes, the pads, and all other instruments which one applies to the fractures to hold the member in straight position and painlessly glossocomes, that is to say, engines or machines, which one applies to hold the member in one position without the patient's being able to move it to right or to left, high or low, whether awake or sleeping, as much as is possible for him. Further, every time the patient is treated, the surgeon will consider diligently whether the bone is in its true position and situation and, if it should not be, he will make it his duty to put it back.

On the manner of treating fractures of the bones with wound. Chapter 11.

Having heretofore amply discoursed on the simple fractures of the bones, subsequently it behooves to discuss the manner by which a compound fracture is to be treated, that is to say, with wound. In order to show this more evidently, we shall take for example a leg of which the two fociles will be entirely broken with wound. This happened to me the fourth day of the month of May, 1561, as Monsieur Nestor, doctor regent in the Faculty of Medicine, Richard Hubert and Antoine Portail, master barber surgeons at Paris, whose renown is sufficiently known, will be amply able to testify, being summoned and I with them, to visit some patients in the village of Les Bons Hommes near Paris.

The misfortune befell me in the manner which follows: Wishing to pass across the water and trying to make my hackney enter a boat, I struck her on the crupper with a riding crop, stimulated by which the animal gave me such a kick that she broke entirely the two bones of my left leg at four inches above the juncture of the foot. Having received the blow and fearing that the horse might kick again, I stepped back one pace, and suddenly fell to the ground; the already fractured bones came out, and broke the flesh, the hose, and the boot, whence I felt such pain that it is not possible for a man (at least according to my judgment) to endure greater without death. My bones thus broken and my foot bent upward, I feared greatly that my leg had to be cut off to save my life. Therefore, casting my sight and my mind to heaven, I invoked the name of God and prayed Him that it might please Him of His benign grace to assist me in this extreme necessity.

I was quickly carried into the boat to cross to the other side in order to have me treated. But its shaking almost made me die, because the ends of the broken bones rubbed against the flesh, and those who were carrying me could not give it fit posture. From the boat I was carried into a house of the village with greater pain than I had endured in the boat, for one held my body, another my leg, the other my foot, and in walking one lifted to the left, the other lowered to the right. Finally, however, they placed me on a bed to regain my breath a little, where, while my dressing was being made, I had my whole body wiped dry, because I was in a general sweat. If I had been thrown in the water, I would not have been wetter. This done, I was treated with a medicament such as we were able to practice in the said place, which we compounded of white of eggs, wheat flour, oven soot, with fresh melted butter.

Above all, I prayed M. Richard Hubert not to spare me any more than if I had been the greatest stranger in the world as far as he was concerned, and that in reducing the fracture he put in oblivion the friendship that he bore me. Further, I admonished him, although he knew his art perfectly, to put my foot strongly in a straight line, and that if the wound were not sufficient in size, that he should increase it with a razor in order more easily to put the bones back in their natural position. Also, that he should search diligently in the wound with his fingers, rather than with another instrument (for the sense of feeling is more certain than any other instrument), in order to take out the fragments and pieces of bones which could be separated from their whole, and especially that he should express and make issue forth the blood which was in great abundance around the wound.

Having done this, that he should begin to bandage the wound and make three or four turns upon it, pressing it rather moderately, in order to express entirely the blood contained in the part; then that he should guide the rest of the bandage to near the knee, in order to prevent the blood and the humors from flowing back into the wound. Afterward that he should have a second bandage which would begin again on the wound one turn or two, which thereafter would be directed, tightening a little more, as far as on the foot in order to end there. Besides this, that he should take a third one and should begin his bandage on the foot, guiding it to the opposite of the first, so that its revolutions might be a little distant from each other and end at the same place as the first, in order that the muscles which had been in any way twisted by the first bandage and changed from their natural position might be put back in it. The leg thus bandaged will be placed in such a position as we have said. Then will be applied to it lengthwise a few splints or ferules, named by the Greeks splenia, two or three fingers wide, and as long as will be needed in order that they may aid to hold the bones in their natural position. Also, it behooves to put the splints far from each other by two fingers or about, especially to bend them a bit in order to lie better on the roundness of the member and to make them less broad at the ends, in order that they may compress the part better. These splints will be compressed and bound with small ribbons of thread, similar to those with which women wind their hair, and they will be tighter at the place of the fracture than in the other places. After the splints pads of straw will be applied, in which it will be necessary to put rather slender and strong sticks to hold the straw firm and stiff. Also, it will be necessary to wrap the pads in a linen cloth and to put them to the right and left of the broken member to hold it in a straight position. Finally, to place it on a small cushion as you see in this figure:

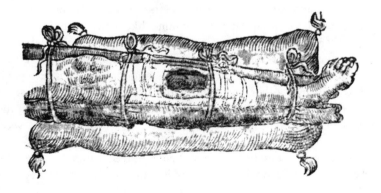

And there is no doubt that it is necessary to bandage over the wound, otherwise it would swell as receiving the humors from the other parts, whence many complications would occur. As one can see, if some fleshy and quite healthy part is bandaged only above and below without including the middle, the part not compressed will swell greatly, as we see by experience, and will change color, becoming livid because of the too great multitude of humors which are sent from the surrounding pressed parts. By stronger reason, such a thing will be done if the part is ulcerated, seeing that without ulcer or wound such a thing is done. For these causes, the ulcer is rendered insuppurative and lachrymose, that is to say that from it distils an unsavory and clear discharge, as are the tears which drip from the eyes when they are injured by inflammation. Now, if this unsavory humor flows and remains long on the substance of the bones, it alters and rots them, even sooner if they are thin and soft than if they are more solid and hard. This alteration and putrefaction would never occur if the patient were well bandaged and dressed. For this, I warn the surgeon not to fail to bandage on the wound if it is possible, that is to say, if there is not so great a pain and inflammation that it might hinder doing this. For then one would be forced to leave the proper treatment in order to relieve the complication, for the care of which there will be taken a cloth folded in two or three doubles, then in the fashion of a large compress, of such width that it can cover and compress the wound with a single revolution, it will be applied thereon, for making it too narrow (as says Hippocrates)* it squeezes the wound like a belt, pressing it unevenly. By this it causes pain, inflammation, and other complications because of the humors which are attracted into it. However, it is always necessary to press and tighten on the wound less than in another part. The cloth will be attached and sewn at the side of the wound, and when one wishes to treat the patient, it will be necessary to unsew it without in any way, if it is possible, moving and shaking the fractured bones. For the fracture does not demand being moved often, as does the wound, in order to be dressed as is required. It is necessary also

---

*Hippocrates, *On Fractures*

that the pads of straw compress from the hip to the extremity of the foot and that the sides of the fracture be somewhat compressed by these with compresses. Likewise, some compresses will be put under the knee joint and near the heel in order to fill these hollow parts, in order that all parts of the leg be supported evenly and smoothly. Of all of this, nothing must be forgotten.

How the author was treated, having been carried to his dwelling after the first dressing. Chapter 13.

My leg treated thoroughly in the aforesaid manner, after dinner I was carried to my dwelling, where I had three saucers of blood drawn from my left basilic vein. At the second dressing and others following, I was cared for by my companion surgeons of Paris, principally by Master Estienne de la Riviere, surgeon ordinary of the King, who took the principal charge of treating me.

Around the wound and neighboring parts, I had rose ointment applied, which was continued until the abscess and suppuration occurred. The compresses and bandages were steeped in oxycrate, sometimes in thick and astringent wine to strengthen the part, to hold back and drive in the humors, and when they were dry I had them moistened with the oxycrate, for when they are too dry, pain and inflammation occur in the part because they compress the member more than they did when wet. There are many surgeons who in such case use only astringent and adhesive medicaments in opposition to Hippocrates and Galen, considering that their astriction and adhesiveness stop up the pores of the skin of the part. Doing this, they increase the foreign warmth with a great pruritus or itching, by means of which is formed beneath the skin a certain serous, acrid, and mordant humidity which makes ulcers, which shows clearly that such medicaments are not to be continued long. Rather, in their place, it is necessary to apply rose ointment which moderates the foreign warmth, prevents the pruritus, and appeases the pain.

And to return to my purpose, I kept at the beginning of my malady such an extreme diet that for the space of nine days I ate each day only twelve Damascus plums, six pieces of bread, and drank a pint of water hippocras, made in this way:

℞ of whitest sugar ℥ xii, of spring water lb. xii, of cinnamon ℥ iii; let them boil together according to the art.

At other times of the syrup of Venus's-hair, with cooked water, at other times of the divine potion, made thus:

℞ of cooked water lb. vi, of whitest sugar ℥ iiii, of juice of lemon ℥ i. Let it all be beaten together in two ewers of glass or other vessels, to use it. At times also, I used a bolus of cassia with a little rhubarb, at other times suppository of soap, to provoke my bowels, a thing which I feared a great deal because it was necessary to move me in order to put a doubled cloth under me, besides the fact that when I was some time without going there I felt great warmth in my kidneys.

There was not, however, so exquisite a regimen nor other things which might keep the fever from seizing me the eleventh day with a discharge and abscess which suppurated a long time. All of this I believe happened to me because of some humor retained in the part, as well as for not having known how to endure the wound's being bandaged, especially because of several splinters comminuted and separated from the ends of the bones while reducing the fracture, for the ends of the one and of the other part were not equal. When there are several small fragments of the whole separated, they cannot be united or agglutinated any more. Therefore, they are altered and rot. This is often the cause of making abscesses and other great complications. Now the signs which caused me to recognize that there were separated bones were that from the wound issued a clear and unsavory discharge. Likewise, the lips of the ulcer were very swollen and the flesh lax and soft as a sponge. Beyond which causes, it seems to me that the principal occasion of the fever and of the abscess arose from the fact that one night, while I was sleeping, my muscles drew back with so great a violence that I raised my leg in the air, indeed in such a way that the bones came out of their position and pressed the lips of the wound so that it was necessary again to pull my foot to reduce them. In doing this, I endured even more pain than I had done the first time that I was treated.

On the cause of tremors in fractured members. Chapter 14.

I do not wish to forget to say what I believe about the contraction and tremors of the muscles which in sleeping occur in fractures. The cause, in my opinion, is that in sleeping the natural warmth, withdrawing to the center of our body, causes the extremities to remain chilled. Whence it comes about that nature, wishing by its accustomed providence to send some spirits in order to succor the wounded part and not finding it disposed to receive them, permits them to withdraw suddenly to the inside whence they were sent. The muscles likewise pull the bones to which they are attached and, making this contraction, take them away from their position with very great pain. As for the fever, it continued in me for seven days, at the end of which it was ended, part by the abscess and part by very great sweats.

Warning for the position of the heel. Chapter 15.

It must be noted here that if the heel in such fractures is not well placed, the patient will be forever lame, for if it is placed too high, the fracture will remain more concave than it should. On the contrary, if it is held lower than is necessary and badly sustained or supported, the bones will remain convex and gibbous in the anterior part. For this, it is expedient to give it the best care that one can. Whatever thing that one may do it, still the fact is that the patient, being for such a long time couched on his back (without being in any way able to move except with an extreme pain in the fracture), the heel, the back, and principally the os sacrum or rump, and, generally, all the muscles of the thigh and of the leg cause extreme pains, because the parts remaining in tension without their accustomed movements are warmed by a non-natural warmth and are put to sleep and made numb because of the too-long tension and compression, whence arise discharge and abscess, then ulcers, principally on the rump, because this part is little fleshy, rather, is membranous and cartilaginous. The heel, similarly, which is very sensitive because of the great tendon (which surrounds and covers it, made of the three muscles of the calf of the leg and of the nerves which pass at its sides), is subject to similar misfortunes, and the ulcers in such parts are difficult to cure, for often caries and corruption are made, from which one has seen ensue continued fever, delirium, spasm, and singultus, because of the nerves of the sixth conjugation which are distributed to the stomach, and of those which are disseminated

79

and spread in the muscles serving the respiration. All of these complications caused the patient to die in a few days, as much because the inflammation and the putrid vapors were communicated to the noble parts by the veins, arteries, and nerves, as because the respiration and inspiration failed. Considering all these things, I often had my heel and lower back raised, but quite gently for fear of shaking and removing from their place the fractured bones, in order to give transpiration and expiration of the parts. Likewise, I had a pad put under my buttocks, of round figure, filled with down, in order that my rump should be supported in the air and not touch anything. Also, I had another small one put under my heel, continuing always the application of the rose ointment to remedy the warmth and pain of the whole leg.

On the remedies proper for the ulcer. Chapter 16.

As for the particular remedies of the ulcer, I had applied on it a suppurative made of the yellow of eggs, of common oil, and of turpentine with a little wheat flour. Then some time afterward, in order to cleanse and heal the ulcer, I used such a medicament:

℞ of rose syrup, of Venice turpentine, of each ℥ ii, of powder of root of Florentine iris, of aloes, of mastic, of barley flour, of each ℨ ss. Let all be incorporated together, let cleanser be made.

And as for the place where I had conjectured the bones were to come out, I had tents of sponge and others put in it, and within the depth of the ulcer catagmatic cephalic powders with a little cooked alum in order to make the fragments of the separated bones come out. When these were out, the ulcer was cured and cicatrized with cooked alum which, having desiccative and astringent virtue, renders the flesh that is soft and spongy and drenched with superfluous humidity firm and hard and finally aids nature to form the skin and the cicatrix. To make the callus, this plaster was used, which I had many times used in similar cases, finding in it great and marvelous effects, because it causes no inflammation or pruritus and also because it dries and astricts moderately, as one can recognize by its ingredients:

℞ of oil of myrtle and of roses, of verjuice, of each lb. ss, of juice of root of althea lb. ii, of root of ashtree and of its leaves, of root of greater comfrey and its leaves, of leaves of willow, of each m. i. Let decoction be made in sufficient quantity of black wine and forge water to half consumption, in the straining add powder of myrrh and of frankincense, of each ℥ ss, of goat fat lb. ss, of washed turpentine ℥ iiii, of mastic ℥ iii, of litharge of gold and of silver, of each ℥ ii, of Armenian bole and of sealed earth, of each ℥ i ss, of minium ℥ vi, of white wax as much as suffices. Let plaster be made as the art teaches. In place of this one can use the black plaster composed in this manner:

℞ of litharge of gold lb. i, of oil and of vinegar lb. ii ss. Let them be cooked together on a slow fire until a black and shining plaster is formed and it does not adhere to the fingers.

Or this one:

℞ of rose oil, of myrtle, of each ℥ ii, of cypress nuts, of Armenian bole, of dragon's blood, pulverized, of each ℥ ss, of plaster of diacalcytheos ℥ iiii. Let them be liquefied together, and let plaster be made according to the art. And, in default of these, it is necessary to use sparadrap, of which here is the composition:

℞ of powder of frankincense, of volatile flour, of mastic, of Armenian bole, of pine resin, of cypress nuts, of dyer's madder [garance], of each ℥ ii, of sheep's fat, of white wax, of each lb. ss. Let plaster be made, in which one is to plunge, while it is warm, some rather worn cloth to use it as above. In such treatments it will always be necessary to pay heed to the temperament of the body, for no one suspects (if he is not indeed deprived of reason) that it is as necessary to dry a young child as it is an old man. Because if one used as desiccative medicaments on a child as one would do for an old man, one would consume the humor of which the callus is to be made. Therefore, it is necessary for the surgeon to look well at such a thing. For, however good and laudable the remedies are, nevertheless for being indiscreetly applied there often occur very pernicious complications for which one can accuse the surgeon who has not conducted his work by reasonable method, as it appears when the callus is made too soft, too large, too small, twisted or too late.

By what signs one will recognize the callus to be made.
Chapter 17.

Veritably, I recognized that the callus was beginning to be made in my fracture when the ulcer began to cast out less discharge than usual, when the pains ceased and, similarly, the contractions of the muscles and tremors, which was the cause that I did not wish to have my leg dressed as often as I did before. For in wiping the wound when the callus is being made, one dries the ros, cambium, and gluten, which are the proper aliment of the substance of the bone as well as of the flesh. I recognized it also, because around the wound one saw issue from the pores a small sanguinolent sweat which stained the compresses and bands. This occurs because, the matter of the callus amassed in this place, nature pushes out by the porosities of the skin some sanguinolent dew in the manner of perspiration. Then I felt a vapor or exhalation with a small tempered warmth which proceeded from the upper parts as far as the wound, withal, a feeling which was very agreeable.

Then I did not wish any longer to hold the part so compressed, for fear of preventing the descent of the matter of the callus, and I began to use foods proper for forming a gross and viscous sap, which easily is transformed into the substance of the callus, as are the tendinous and cartilaginous extremities of animals, that is, legs, knuckles, and feet of ox, snouts and ears of pig, heads of kid, of calf, of sheep, and of lamb, which were cooked most often with rice or hulled barley, diversifying them today with one and tomorrow with the other. I also used frumenty or panada of pure wheat bread. I drank rather thick claret wine, moderately diluted. These foods are first received in the stomach, in which they are prepared, then sent to the intestines, from which they are attracted to the mesenteric veins, and from these to the portal vein, from it to the liver, then to the great hollow vein, and from there into the veins which are distributed through the whole body, of which some especially carry the blood in the bones in which the marrow is made, which is the proper nourishment of these. For this reason, it is contained in the cavity of the great bones and in the small cavities and porosities of the small bones, in which there is a humor which is propitious nourishment for them in place of the said marrow.

Now, the marrow is formed in the thickest part of the blood, which is carried to the cavities of the great bones by great veins and arteries, and to the small by small ones which end in the porosities of these. But in the great bones, one finds manifest cavities through which the said veins and arteries enter, for the same causes as above. Likewise, also, nerves enter there from which is made a membrane which envelopes and covers the said marrow. By means of this, the said membrane has excellent feeling, as experience shows, not that I wish to say that the medulla of itself has feeling, rather only its membrane. From this medulla is made a crass and earthy sweat from which the callus is formed and made by the nutritive virtue, holding the place of the formative virtue. Of the time of this callus a definite rule cannot be given, as we have said above, because the things which prevent its generation are taken away sooner from some and later from others.

On the remedies which aid to make the callus. Chapter 18.

After having thus declared the signs by which one will recognize the beginning of the callus, its generation, and the manner by which it is made, now it behooves to say what prevents the generation of the said callus and what aids nature to form and harden it. Now, the things which prevent the callus from being made, or which delay it, are all unctuous, oleaginous, humid, and resolvent things. For by these is softened, relaxed, subtilized, liquefied, and consumed the humor of which it is to be made, which, contrarily, one is to dry, enlarge, thicken, and harden with emplastic, warm, and astringent medicaments. Yet I do not wish to deny that the humid and relaxing medicaments should be used where the callus would be too thick or twisted or of other bad figure, in order to diminish it and break it anew, which is done when the part is greatly deformed and its action marred, provided that it is still recent. This one will do with fomentations of decoctions of tripes and heads of sheep, in which one will cook roots of marshmallow, bryony, flax seed, fenugreek, pigeon dung, laurel seed, and others similar. Also it will be necessary to use this liniment and plaster:

℞ of ointment of dialthea ℥ iiii, of oil of lilies, of goosefat, of each ℥ i, of brandy a little; let them be liquefied together, let liniment be made with which the part is to be rubbed. Then put on this plaster:

℞ of Vigo's plaster with mercury, of cerate of hyssop, descriptione filagri, of each ℥ iii, of oil of dill and of lilies, of each ℥ i. Let all be liquefied together; let plaster be made, let it be spread on soft leather for the use said.

The callus being rather softened, it is necessary to break it and straighten the bones in their natural figure and to practice all the things necessary to perfect the cure. If the callus is too hardened and old, it is better not to try to break it, rather to leave it for fear of doing worse to the patient. For it can happen that if one tries to break and rend it, the bone will sooner break in another place than in the place of the callus. Therefore, the patient will be wiser to be content to live being crippled than to put himself back into the hands of such menders in order to make himself die miserably. If the callus was not twisted or of other bad figure, but only too thick, one will diminish it, at least if it is recent, by soothing and resolvent medicaments which liquefy, consume, and dry. Similarly, it will be good to rub it often and long with laurel oil in which one will dissolve saltpeter or other salt, and the swelling will be bandaged rather tightly with a plate of lead.

If the callus is sometimes too small and delayed in being made because the bandages are too tight and the part has been long at rest without any exercise (which is one of the principal causes of rendering it emaciated), considering that movement warms the part, by which it is better nourished and consequently stronger, or if the retardation comes by fault of foods failing in quality or in quantity, or in both together, one will obviate these vices by administering to the patient the drink and food written above, for the generation of the callus. If it is for having compressed the part too much, it will be necessary to loosen it and to remove the bandage wholly from above the fracture, in place of which will be made another manner of binding, which will begin at the root of the vessels, that is, near the groin, guiding it as far as near the fracture. By this means, one expresses the blood and makes it flow to the injured part, just as heretofore we have done the contrary to drive the blood from the part. Likewise, one can use soft frictions and fomentations with warm water, which it will be necessary to leave off when one sees some warmth and swelling in the part. For if one continued further, one would resolve what one would have drawn to it. Simple fractures of the leg are most often agglutinated by the callus in forty days.

Because of the wound and of the separated splinters and other complications which were in my leg, I was two months and more before the callus was made, during which I remained always on my back (which is a species of Gehenna to a poor patient). I was yet another month before I could even press my foot on the ground without a crutch, which I began to do with pains, for the reason that the callus held the place of the muscles and that the cicatrix of the ulcer did not permit the extension and flexion of the muscles. For before the movement can be free, it is necessary that little by little the tendons and membranes be separated or loosened from against the cicatrix. Yet, thanks to God, I have been entirely cured without limping in any fashion. On this, I shall make an end of the treatise on fractures and shall pray God that He will to guard from such an accident all those who will read this history and to send me death rather than to fall into it again, yet may His will be done.

Because in this book we have almost no other subject than the bones, I have wished to draw from my *Universal Anatomy* these two figures of the skeleton or osteotomy, in order to refresh your memory, of which you will have the declaration exposed by letters.

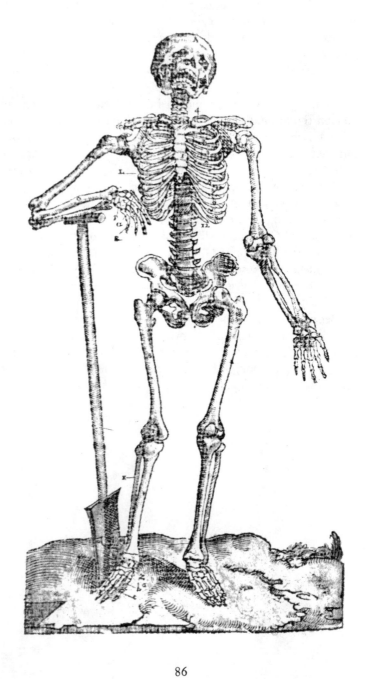

Declaration of the letters of the first figure of the bones.

A. The coronal bone.

B. Two parietal bones, one on each side.

C. Two petrous bones, one on each side.

D. The zygoma.

E. The lower jaw.

F. Right clavicle and the same on the other side.

G. The superior apophysis of the scapula, called acromion.

H. The anterior apophysis of the scapula, named coracoid or crow's beak.

I. The sternum, which receives the seven true ribs.

K. The cartilage named xiphoid, in French "la fourchette" [the fork].

L. The twenty-four ribs, twelve on each side, of which there are seven true and five false, which are marked by 1, 2, 3, 4, 5, 6, 7, etc.

M. The arm or brachium or humerus, commonly the adjutory.

N. The bone of the elbow, commonly called the large focile of the arm.

O. The ray or radius, commonly called the small focile of the arm.

P. The wrist or carpus, composed of eight small bones.

Q. The forehand or metacarpus, containing four bones.

R. The bones of the fingers, three in each side, which make fifteen in all.

S. The bone of the thigh, called femur or crus.

T. The saucer or rotula of the knee, called patella.

V. The bone of the leg, called tibia or large focile of the leg.

X. The spur called perone or fibula, commonly the small focile of the leg.

Y. The astragalus [talus].

Z. The naviform or navicular bone.

a. The four bones of the tarsus.

b. The five bones of the metatarsus.

c. The fourteen bones of the digits, three in each, and two in the big toe.

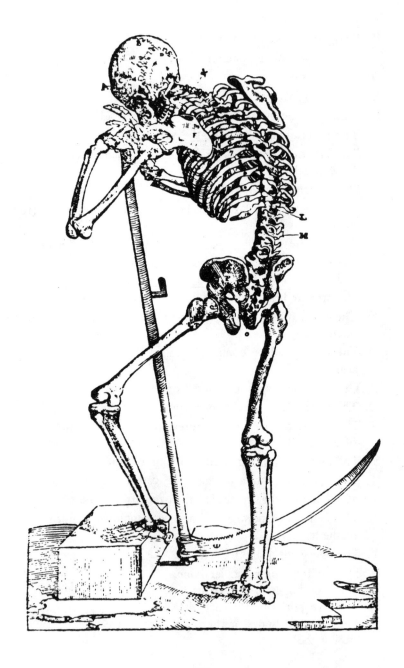

Declaration of the letters of the second figure of the bones.

A. Marks the place of the coronal suture.

B. The sagittal suture.

C. The two false sutures.

D. The lambdoid suture.

E. The occipital bone.

F. The shoulder blade or scapula.

G. The neck of the scapula.

H. The head of the arm [humerus].

I. The tip of the elbow called by the Greeks, olecranon.

K. The seven vertebrae of the neck, and beside a little lower are the ribs marked 1, 2, etc.

L. The twelve thoracic vertebrae.

M. The five of the loins [lumbar vertebrae].

N. The sacrum.

O. The bone of the tail, called the os caude or coccyx.

P. The os amplum or ilium, made in young children of three bones and commonly named by three names. The superior part is called ilium, that which receives the head of the bone ischium, and the anterior part os pubis.

Q. The head of the femur, called vertebrum.

R. The greater trochanter.

T. The lesser trochanter.

V. The calx, calcaneus, or heel.

The Fourth Book

treats of contusions and has 7 *chapters*

TABLE OF THE CHAPTERS OF THE FOURTH BOOK.

On Contusions

Book IV.
On the differences of contusions. Chapter 1.

Now we shall treat of contusions and bruises, which are made in diverse manners, according to the blood, which now spreads out in the interior parts, now in the depth of the body, and sometimes only in the exterior parts. Now, the blood spreads out within the body when, for example, someone falls from the top to the bottom of a breach, or when he has been pressed under some great and heavy burden, as happens in mines in which quite often a great quantity of earth or of stones falls on the soldiers and miners, or by an extreme tension as is that of the rack, or by too much unbridled yelling, by means of which excess some vessel of the lungs can break. Likewise, for an arquebusade received through the body, the blood can come out of the vessels, a part of which is cast out by stools and urines, as I have seen happen to many, especially to the late Monsieur de Martigues, who at the late siege of Hedin, wishing to see by the rampart of the wall the enemy who were sapping it at the foot, was struck through the body by an arquebus shot. Immediately after, he cast out blood by the mouth, by the seat, and the staff, which was the cause of his death.

Further, the blood can spread out in the body as a result of being struck by dry blows, as are those of stick, mace, stone, and, to say in one word, of all things which can contuse, bruise, and make the blood come out of the veins and arteries, which because of this are pressed, expressed, broken, and lacerated. Chiefly, most often the exterior parts of them are also greatly contused and wounded with cut, and sometimes without cut, so that the skin remains quite entire but the blood is spread out in the muscles and between skin and flesh only. This disposition is named by the ancients ecchymosis. Following the difference of these contusions, we will have to diversify the treatment of these, as we shall presently declare.

On the general treatment of great and enormous contusions.
Chapter 2.

The blood which has flowed within the body is to be evacuated palpably or impalpably. Palpable evacuation will be made as much by bleedings, cupping glasses, cornets with scarifications, and leeches, as by medicines proper and dedicated to such a thing, as are the solvents. One will evacuate it impalpably by resolvent potions provoking sweat, or by baths, and by means of the lightest diet.*

This is approved by Hippocrates who says that if someone has fallen from a height, the same day or the next one is to give him a medicine, or a bleeding, not only to purge the superfluous humor but to divert it so that it does not fall to the

---

*On Fractures.

wounded part. Similarly, Galen says that if someone has fallen from a height, even though he might not have enough blood, still some must be drawn from him to obviate its coagulating and putrefying inside, being outside of its proper vessels.

Therefore, the surgeon must not omit drawing blood according to the great vehemence of the ill and the plentitude and strength of the patient. Having done this, he is to give him to drink a draft of oxycrate, which prevents the coagulation of the blood in the stomach, as Galen commands, and then to envelope him in a recently flayed sheep skin, on which will be spread powder of myrtle, of nasturtium, and of finely pulverized salt. One will then place him on his bed where, being well covered, he will sweat quite at his ease. The next day, it will be necessary to take away the skin and anoint him with the liniment which follows, which appeases pain and dissolves the bruised blood:

℞ of ointment of dialthea ℥ vi, of oil of earthworms, of camomile, of dill, of each ℥ ii, of Venice turpentine ℥ iiii, of flour of fenugreek, of pulverized red roses, of powder of myrtle, of each ℥ i. Let litus be made for the use said.

Likewise, one will give him to drink the following potion, which provokes sweat and dissolves the blood coagulated within the body:

℞ of wood of guaiac ℥ viii, of root of elecampane, of greater comfrey, of Florentine iris, of polypody of oak, of each ℥ ss, of seed of coriander, of anise, of each ℥ ss, of licorice ℥ ii, of catnip, of centaury, of cloves, of blessed thistle, of verbena, of each m. ss, of spring water lb. xii; all crushed let them be steeped for the space of twelve hours, according to the art let them be cooked on a slow fire to the consumption of half.

When the patient has taken in the morning a half-pint of this potion somewhat tepid, he will let himself sweat for an hour in the bed, more or less each time, and will continue six or seven days as there is need of it. If it were some poor soldier who cannot have such conveniences, it will behoove to put him in some manure, enveloping him first in a cloth and putting on him a little hay, or white straw, before burying him in the manure up to the throat, and to keep him there until one sees that he has sweated enough. This I have done many times. Likewise, one will give the patient some syrups to drink which are proper for preventing the coagulation and putrefaction of the blood, as acetous syrups, of lemons, or of the sourness of lemons, the quantity of an ounce dissolved in water of scabious or of holy thistle for each time. Also, one is to give promptly this potion, which is proper for keeping the blood from coagulating and which likewise comforts the internal parts:

℞ of selected rhubarb pulverized ℥ i, of water of red madder and plantain, of each ℥ i, of theriac ℨ ss, of syrup of dry roses ℥ ss, let a potion be made.

This will be given to the patient immediately and repeated for four or five mornings. Or, in its place, one will have him drink a dram of spermaceti dissolved with water of bugloss, or of the waters written above, with one ounce, or a half-ounce of syrup of Venus's-hair.

After the use of the said potion it will behoove to have the patient take for the space of nine days, in the morning two or three hours before his meal, the powder which follows, if it is necessary:

℞ of rub. torref., of root of red madder, of centaury, of gentian, of round birthwort, of each ℥ ss.

This will be given each time one dram with acetous syrup and water of holy thistle.

Further, the water of green nuts, drawn in alembic and drunk, has great virtue of dissolving amassed and coagulated blood.

One can likewise use baths made with decoction of root of iris, of elecampane, of sorrel, of butcher's broom, of fennel, of althea, of water fern, of greater comfrey, of seed of fenu-greek, of sage leaves, of marjoram, of flowers of camomile, of melilot, and their like.

Also, the seeds found under the hay have great efficacy to this same end.

The bath in temperate warmth has this utility, that it loosens and makes thin the skin, melts and dissolves the ac-cumulated blood, cuts the viscid humors, sweetens the sour, and draws them from the depth of the body to the surface of the skin, so that one part of them is voided by a general sweat, another by spitting and blowing the nose, if perchance the affection is in the superior parts; by the stool and urine, if it is in the inferior. Baths also are profitable to inflammations of the lungs, to the pleuritic, because they appease the pain and help to suppurate and cast out by the spittle the superfluities contained in the said parts. They can likewise aid in several other dispositions, provided that they be made duly after the general things. For, if they were administered before the bleeding and purgation, they would harm greatly, for the reason that they could cause new discharge in the injured parts. Therefore, I advise you always to use the counsel of the learned and expert physician, if it is possible for you.

On the manner of treating contusions with wound. Chapter 3.

If the contusion is with wound, it is necessary at the beginning to prevent the defluxion with ointment of bole, whites of eggs, of rose oil, of myrtle, of powder of red roses, of alum, and of mastic. And at the second dressing one will use the digestive made with yellow of egg and violet oil with a little turpentine. One can also put on the neighboring parts to aid to suppurate the cataplasm which follows:

℞ of root of althea and of lilies, of each ℥ iiii, of leaves of mallows, of violets, of groundsel, of each m. ss. Let them be cooked complete and let them be passed through setaceum, adding of fresh butter and of violet oil, of each ℥ iii, of volatile flour as much as suffices, let cataplasm be made in the form of a fairly liquid poultice or others similar, in the application of which you will be careful because if they are unduly applied, they render phlegmonous wounds necrotic and putrid. Then, after the suppuration is made, the wound will be cleansed and the flesh regenerated, then led to cicatrix. However, if the contused flesh is greatly lacerated and destituted of its natural warmth, it will be wise to amputate it. But if there is still hope that it can agglutinate itself without cutting, it will be sewn as the thing requires, and the stitches will not be as tight as if it were a simple wound without contusion because such wounds are inflamed and will swell, which would be the cause of lacerating the whole skin with the flesh and of breaking of the stitches.

On contusions without wound. Chapter 4.

Now, if there is no wound which appears and the skin remains whole, the parts beneath remaining contused, and there is effusion of blood under the skin, such disposition (as we have said) is named by the ancients ecchymosis. For the cure of this it is necessary to hold good regimen until the complications have passed.

At the beginning, blood will be drawn from the opposite part, if there is need of it, as much for the evacuation as for the revulsion. Likewise, scarifications will be made on the contusion, and then one will apply cupping glasses or cornets as much to void the blood which makes swelling and tension in the part as to give air to the inflammation, for fear an abscess may be made and other bad complications. Also it is necessary to purge the stomach as one will see it to be necessary. And for the topical and particular remedies, at the beginning it is necessary to use strong and astringent remedies in order to compress the veins and arteries in order to strengthen the part and prevent the defluxion, as can be this which I ordinarily use:

℞ of whites of eggs, three in number, of oil of myrtle and of roses, of each ℥ i, of Armenian bole, of dragon's blood, of each ℥ ss, of nuts of cypress, of galls, of powder of burnt alum an. ℨ ii. Let all be incorporated, adding a little vinegar, and let medicine be made.

Then one will use fomentations, cataplasms, and resolvent plasters.

On the means of obviating the menaces of the gangrenes which can follow contusions. Chapter 5.

Great contusions are dangerous, for by these occur sometimes gangrenes and mortifications. Now, when the part is very black and livid to the point of seeming that it is dead and its warmth almost extinct because of the great concretion of the blood which has flowed into it, then one is, to void and discharge the part, to apply cupping glasses or cornets, having first scarified the part with a razor, lancets, or small lancets, as you see in this figure:

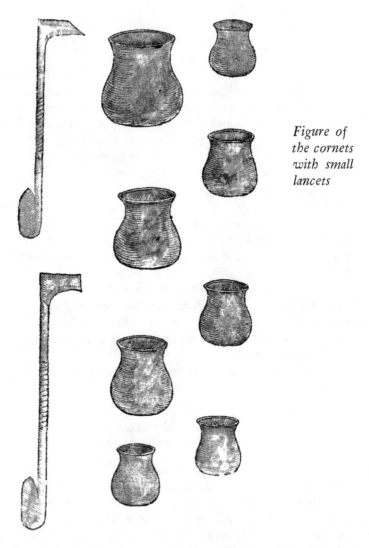

Figure of the cornets with small lancets

Or else with the instrument called scarifier, which you also see figured here, within which are inserted eighteen wheels cutting as a razor, marked FFF, which one tightens with a spring marked C and are released by another marked D, with which, when you wish to make several scarifications to evacuate the blood spread out beneath the skin, you will be able to aid yourself more promptly and with less pain, for the reason that eighteen incisions are as quickly made as a single one.

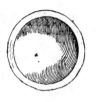

b. shows the box.
a. the cover.

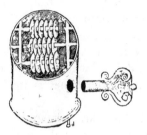

Instrument called scarifier.

Then one is to foment the part with strong vinegar in which one will have boiled roots of radish, or of greater dragonwort, arum, or Solomon's seal, orpiment, and others similar. Such acrid things warm strongly, separate, resolve, and attract the bruised blood from the depth to the surface. This, nevertheless, you will use with discretion for fear of attracting not only the blood which is outside the veins but also that which is contained in them. Likewise, you will use them only when the flow has been completely stopped.

To small bruises one will apply only virgin wax melted with powder of cumin and cloves and a little root of Mary's seal, which in such case has great power of destroying and of promptly resolving all ecchymoses and bruises. Also, one can apply absinthe, crushed a little and heated on a warm iron pan, and sprinkle it with a little white wine or have it fried in a frying pan with wine, oil of camomile, a little wheat bran, powder of clove and nutmeg, adding at the end a little brandy. Then put it between two delicate linens and apply it rather warm to the part. Likewise, the plaster which follows is very resolvent of bruised blood:

℞ of black pitch ʒ ii, of gum elemi ℥ i, of liquid storax and of common turpentine, of each ℥ ss, of powder of live sulphur ℥ i. Let them be liquefied together; let plaster be made; let it be spread on soft leather.

97

Marvelous complication which comes to contusions made on the ribs. Chapter 6.

Sometimes by a great contusion the contused flesh becomes slimy and puffed up, as if one had blown it up with wind, the skin remaining intact, which is seen principally on the ribs*. When one presses on it with the hand, one feels the air which departs with a small whistling, and the impression of the fingers remain, as in edemas. So if one does not give good attention to it, for the reason that the flesh is not attached to the bones, pus is amassed in it which comes to occupy the empty space, and alteration of the bones is made, as one sees occur most often.

For the cure of this slimy swelling, it is necessary to compress and bind the part as strongly as the patient can endure, still leaving his respiration the freest possible, if it is in the thorax. Then there will be applied on the part a plaster of oxycroceum or of diachylon ireatum, mixed with plaster of melilot and resolvent fomentations.

Now, the cause of such swelling is a slimy mucus, which is made by default of good concoction in the part and of half-cooked aliment, as one sees often the conjunctiva of the eye, following a contusion, swell so strongly that it comes out of the cavity of the eye, because the concoctive virtue of the part is weak because of the immoderate temperature or of the humor which flows into it, as one sees in edematic swellings.

Digression of the author touching the use of mummy. Chapter 7.

And it is not to be marveled at if in this treatise of contusions I have made no mention of mummy for giving to the patients to drink, as most do. I can assure you that it is because one does not in truth know what it is, except a rotten flesh of dead men, of bad taste and odor. In this I have found no effect except that it provokes vomiting and wounds the stomach strongly. Because of this, I cannot in conscience and dare not prescribe it for anyone whatsoever.

End of the fourth book.

---

*Hippocrates, *On Fractures*

CRÜJÜRÜJÜRÜJÜRÜJÜRÜJÜRÜJÜRÜJÜRÜJÜRÜJÜRÜJÜRÜJÜRÜ

The Fifth Book

treats of the method of dressing burns resulting principally from cannon powder and contains four chapters.

TABLE OF THE CHAPTERS OF THE BOOK OF BURNS.

The Method

of treating burns made principally by cannon powder.

Book V.

On the difference in burns. Chapter 1.

Burns made by cannon powder or metals, oil, water, fire,
or other materials differ only in the degree of the burn.

The action of fire in producing a burn leaves damaging heat
in the part, condenses the skin, rendering it hard, and produces
great pain. It is the cause of attracting humors from the parts
near and distant, converting them into serous accumulation,
causing blisters. It is necessary to open these as soon as they
are raised, because the humor retained in them acquires an
acrimony, corrodes and dissolves the flesh, causing hollow ulcers.
Thus, by the multiplication of cause and increase of matter, the

inflammation is augmented, not only nine days, according to the common idea, but sometimes longer, sometimes less, according to individual variation, which is until the pain be quieted and the discharge arrested. Then we are to extinguish carefully the remainder of warmth or fieriness left by the action of the fire impressed in the burnt part. A most particular remedy preventing vesication (of which I have several times made experiment) is the immediate application, in the first dressing and no more, of raw onions crushed and beaten with a little salt. And it is to be noted that this remedy has no place except in burns which are not yet excoriated or ulcerated, for it would cause great pain, which it does not do where the skin has remained intact, but rather prevents any furuncles or blisters.

As for the surrounding parts, it is useful to apply cold and repellent medicaments such as litharge ointment, called nutritive, or of bole, and others of similar action. I know that many who have not experimented with the remedy of onions, having considered their warm quality, will condemn their application, wishing to maintain that maladies are cured by their opposites and that a burn is made by heat, wherefore its cure requires cold remedies.

Apparent proof of the value of onions in the first dressing of burns. Chapter 2.

Onions, as Galen says, are warm to the fourth order or degree, whence they are far from opposing burns, but rather they ought to be the cause of increasing them; therefore, they can not fittingly be applied. In spite of the fact that such reasoning has some appearance of probability, still experience, reason, and authority show us the contrary. First, I have seen by experience the said onions do marvels, especially when I treated many soldiers in Piedmont who were burned by a train of cannon powder made by the enemy in the assault on the castle of Villaine. And I can assure you that where I could apply onions in the manner aforesaid, they developed no blisters or pustules, as happened to others to whom the said remedy was not applied. And by reason it can be proved that onions are warm potentially and humid actually. Thus, by their warm temperature they rarefy and by the actual humidity relax the skin. By this same means they attract, consume, drain, and dry the already inflamed humor and doing this they prevent blistering. We see this daily in those who burn their fingers, for almost by their natural instinct they are taught to bring them near the fire and warm them well, in such manner that by such warmth they prevent vesication. Which it seems should not be more remarkable to us than the consideration of poisonous beasts, which because of the antagonism that they have with our body in all their substance, by a single bite, or by very little of their saliva, in brief time take away our life. In the treatment of this hazard no surer and better remedy has been invented than to take these beasts, crush them, and apply them to the wound, to the place where they have impressed their virulent saliva. These are rather occult things and not subject to reason. For this cause we esteem a sovereign aid to those wounded by the crocodile or lizard to apply to the wound immediately the fat of the said lizard or crocodile. Similarly, for those who have been bitten or stung by a scorpion or spider, these beasts crushed and applied, as is said, are a sovereign remedy, which Galen teaches us in his book *De theriaca ad Pisionem.*

By authority Galen persuades me in the fifth book *Of Simples* that maladies are not always cured by contrary qualities but sometimes by similar, although any cure may be made by opposites, taking opposites broadly. This manifestly appears in phlegmons, which are often cured by warm resolvent medicaments, which, by evacuating the matter, cures them. Wherefore I dare conclude the application of onions, as has been said, to be beneficial in the early treatment of burns.

How burns must be treated after the first dressing.
Chapter 3.

Having used the remedy above for the first dressing, it is not necessary to continue it in the second and following, but the ointment called nutritive is useful in removing warm intemperature, principally dispensed in the following form:

℞ of litharge of gold ℥ iiii, of rose oil ℥ iii, of oil of poppy ℥ ii ss, of water of nightshade and of plantain, of each ℥ ii, of populeon ointment ℥ iiii, of camphor ℨ i. Let ointment be made in a leaden mortar according to the art. And where there might be blisters, it would be necessary to cut them at once and on the excoriations use the ointment which follows:

℞ of fresh butter, without salt, burnt and strained ℥ vi, yolks of four eggs, of ceruse washed in water of plantain ℥ ss, of tutty similarly washed ʒ iii, of burnt and washed lead ʒ ii. Let all be mixed together; let liniment be made as is fitting. And it is necessary to increase or diminish the dryness according to the nature of the ulcer.

Another:

℞ of Rhazes's white ointment, camphorated, and of rose ointment, of each ℥ iii. Let them be mixed together, let ointment be made.

Another:

℞ of bark of green elder and of oil of roses, of each lb. i. Let them boil together on a slow fire, then let them be strained and add of oil of eggs ℥ iiii, of powder of ceruse and of prepared tutty, of each ℥ i, of white wax as much as suffices. Let soft ointment be made according to the art.

Another of similar virtue:

℞ of oil of yolks of eggs ℥ iiii, of oil of poppy ℥ ii, of litharge of gold, of ceruse, of lead burnt and washed, of washed tutty, each ℥ i, of water of plantain, and of nightshade, of each ℥ ii ss, of Rhazes's white populeon ointment, of each ℥ i ss. Let all be mixed in a leaden mortar; let liniment be made as is fitting. The said oil of eggs is made thus:

It is necessary to take forty fresh eggs and have them cooked well in water, then to take the yolks and break them in small pieces, and then put them to cook in a glazed pan, or one of leaded earth, and hold them on a slow fire until one sees that they are converted into a moist mass. Then it is necessary to put them into a press and to express them as one does oil of almonds. This oil quiets pains marvelously and cleanses moderately. Likewise, many approve as an exceptional remedy this one which I have known to be such by experience:

℞ of old lard cut into bits lb. one. Let it be liquefied in water of roses, then let it be strained through thin linen cloth, and cold, let it be washed four times with water of henbane or another of the same kind. Then let be incorporated with it yolks of fresh eggs to the number of eight. Let ointment be made, which it is necessary to spread on a cloth, and apply it on the ulcerated burn, considering carefully whether the said ulcer is purulent and dirty. For then it would be necessary to add powders of mineral ingredients to the said ointments. As for the quantity, I can not describe it without being charged, with those whom Galen says, with shoeing all persons on the same form. So then I leave the quantity of these powders to the prudent conjecture of the surgeon, knowing well that the quantity of the medicaments cannot rationally be described, as much because of the difference in the dispositions as for the temperaments of the bodies and the parts of these, nor also the time of the application, as has been said many times*. The ink with which we write dries quickly if it is dissolved in water, and therefore it is useful for ulcerated burns if it is applied immediately. Of that also a surgeon showed me great esteem, certifying to me that he had experimented with it and that he had made fine cures with it, whence he held the said ink for a great secret.

On the cleansing of ulcers made by burns and on the cicatrization of these. Chapter 4.

Further, where there may be need of cleansing, it will be necessary to use additional detergents, by applying there some of the powders written in the abovesaid ointments.

℞ of rose syrup ℥ iiii, of turpentine washed in water of barley ℥ iii, of washed aloes ℈ ii, of flour of barley ℥ ss. Let all be incorporated together, and let cleanser be made. This done, if one sees that nature tends to cicatrize the ulcer, it is necessary to wash it with water of plantain in which one has boiled a little alum. Or, one will take water in which some chalk has been dissolved, which has previously been washed eight times. Then add to it powder of rind of pomegranate and of rock alum the quantity that the surgeon will see is to be used. After the ablution it is necessary to apply such healing powder:

℞ of prepared tutty, of litharge of gold, of ceruse, of burnt and washed galls, of each one ounce, of which let some be put on the ulcer to cicatrize. One will also be able to use for the same effect and purpose scales of iron, scales of brass, burnt lead, scales of heads of fish, washed and prepared, unripened gall nuts, burnt rinds of pomegranates. These dry greatly and make cicatrixes without stinging, as is described by Master

*Galen, *Of Simples,* bk. IX

Jacques Hollier, doctor in medicine, in his books on the matter of surgery, which he has composed to the great profit and use of all surgeons.

It often comes about that the burn is so great that it has burned the deeper tissues; still the patient does not feel as great pain as that one does whose burn is lesser and more superficial. This is a daily experience noted in those who are cauterized, for straightway after the cauterization they feel only a very little pain, for the reason that this great burn takes away feeling by burning and deadening the sensitive parts. I have seen this often, and even recently in a child aged ten years or about, who had been found in a wood all rigid without any movement or speech, having only a very little respiration. Brought from the wood, he was put near a fire where he was warmed in such a way that the greatest part of one of his legs was burned. Furthermore, at the place of the burn, the scab was so large and hard that it rendered the part without any feeling. Because of this, some had concluded that it was most expedient to cut off the member. I was called for this, and immediately I scarified it with several rather deep incisions and applied thereon unsalted butter with rose oil and yolks of eggs in good quantity to make the scab fall. Above the knee, I put nutritive ointment with compresses and bandages steeped in oxycrate, which I renewed often, in order to prohibit and prevent the flow of the humors which were produced by means of the pain. After the fall of the scab, I applied Rhazes's white ointment and populeon mixed in equal portion and beaten in a lead mortar, with white of eggs, to take away the pain. This having ceased I increased my remedy of desiccant soothing medicaments, which were Armenian bole, powder of rotten oak, tutty, and some others previously described. These I continued until the time that the ulcer was full and ready to cicatrize. Then I washed the said ulcer several times with lime water, using after the ablution the cicatrizative powder described above, so that by these means the child was perfectly cured.

End of the book of burns.

The Sixth Book

teaches the manner of treating caries of the bones and contains 10 chapters.

On the Manner

of treating caries of the bones. Book VI.

Intention of the Author. Chapter 1.

After having discussed the fractures of the bones, we must now speak of the caries and putrefactions which most often occur in them by reason of the abovesaid complications, a treatise very necessary to the surgeon in order to obviate the perils which follow them. Although I have spoken in my book on the wounds of the head, yet it seems to me that it will not be an unfit thing if I write of it again in this present book because someone will be able to use it who does not have the other at his command. Thus the surgeon will not remain without remedy for the treatment of carious bones.

The causes why the bone alters and putrefies. Chapter 2.

The solution of continuity made in bones is named catagma in the sixth book of the *Method* by Galen. Caries are made in them because they are crushed, split, pierced, fractured, luxated, abscessed, and stripped of their flesh. When then there is wasting away of substance of the flesh which covered them, they are altered, and the blood and their proper nourishment is dried by the surrounding air so that the naked bones cannot long endure without altering. Also, when a wound is of long duration, the discharge flowing over it is absorbed into their substance and rots them. Likewise, by the undue application of oils and other humid and suppurative medicaments because they render the wound necrotic and malignant, then the flesh of the neighboring parts is warmed and suppurates, and the pus flowing on the bone inflames it. Because of this, the patient often falls into fevers. To say it briefly, the bones can suffer all the inconveniences with which the flesh is vexed. Therefore, they can decay and putrefy. Moreover, Galen has left us in writing that often the inflammation begins in the bones. On this some will be able to object that the bones cannot have pulsation, seeing that they have no feeling. For the ancients have left in writing* that the pulse signifies move-

---

*Hippocrates, *On ulcers, on fractures, on unnatural tumors*

ment of the arteries with pain. With this I agree, but I answer also that the membrane which covers them and the arteries and nerves which enter their cavities have exquisite feeling and that when the said arteries move, being warmed by the sick bone, they cause such pain in the membrane which envelopes it that the patients say they feel a pulsatile pain in the depth of the bones.

The signs for recognizing the alteration and caries of the bones. Chapter 3.

Alteration and putrefaction of the bones is sometimes apparent to the eye, that is, when the bone is uncovered. For then one sees that there is change from its natural color, when in place of being white, it is found livid, yellowish, or black. Likewise, one recognizes it by the touch of the sound, when one finds in it roughness and unevenness, and in pushing it one enters into its substance, as into a rotten wood, for the healthy bone must be solid and not soft. Nevertheless, a sure rule must not be made from this sign because I have sometimes seen the bone, having been uncovered for a long time, become altered and so hard that the trepan or other instrument could enter it only with difficulty. Also, the alteration and putrefaction can be recognized by the discharge which comes out of the ulcer, which is thinner and clearer than that which flows from an ulcer in the flesh. It is even less viscid and more stinking than that which comes from the flesh, the nerves, the tendons, and the membranes. Further, in the ulcer will be found always some soft, frothy, and spongy flesh. Likewise, the ulcer will be hard to treat and refuse to close and cicatrize, although still by long continuation of desiccative astringent medicaments one may sometimes induce cicatrix in it. But immediately afterward the ulcer opens and is renewed for the reason that nature cannot make good foundation nor engender a laudable flesh on the alteration and caries of the bone, for it is a thing contrary to nature. Therefore, it is to be removed as quickly as possible.

On the means of proceeding to the separation of carious bones. Chapter 4.

Now, it does not suffice for the surgeon to recognize that the bone is altered and corrupted, but it behooves also that he know if the alteration is superficial or deep in order to diversify the medicaments and the instruments and to give drainage to the discharge which can be in the substance of the bone. To do this, it is necessary to separate the altered and rotted bone. The means of doing this is to correct their corruption by cleansing the ulcer in order that the discharge may not fall on the bone and that it may render it humid; likewise, drying it very strongly as much by medicaments as by potential or actual cauteries, for by this means one renders it bloodless, without nourishment and life. This can be shown by the example of trees, from which the leaves fall because the sap, by which they adhere to the branches, is dried. Thus it comes about that the leaves, no longer having any humidity and life, separate from the green and living tree. Thus, consuming the humidity of the bones, one takes away their life, which is cause of making them separate. Because of this, the powders called catagmatics are proper to aid to separate the bone, which may be altered superficially, as this one written by Nicolas Massa:

℞ of roots of iris, of birthwort, of each ℥ i, of centuary ℥ ii, of bark of pine ℥ ss. Mix, and let them be pulverized very finely, and let some of it be put on the altered bone.

Another:

℞ of powder of aloes, of burnt chalk, of pompholix [zinc oxide], of each ℥ ii, of Florentine iris, of round birthwort, of myrrh, of ceruse, of each ℥ i, of powder of burnt oysters ℥ ss. Let them be ground very finely, let powder be made.

This can be applied alone or with honey, and a little brandy. Also, one can apply some of this plaster, which has the faculty of aiding nature to extract the fractured bones and of cleaning the gross and viscid discharge from the ulcers.

℞ of new wax, of pine resin, of gum ammoniac and elemi, of each ℥ vi, of turpentine ℥ iiii, of powder of mastic, of myrrh, of each ℥ ss, of round birthwort, of Florentine iris, of aloes, of opopanax, of euphorbia, of each ℥ i, of oil of rose as much as suffices. Let plaster be made according to the art. Also plaster of betony has similar virtue.

On the instruments proper for separating the caries from the bones. Chapter 5.

And if the alteration cannot be removed by these remedies,

one can use instruments, of which you have here the illustrations, of several different types.

Raspatories which can be inserted one after the other in their handle.

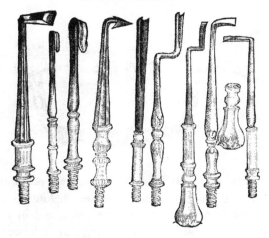

Raspatories of other types than the preceding to cut the bone further.

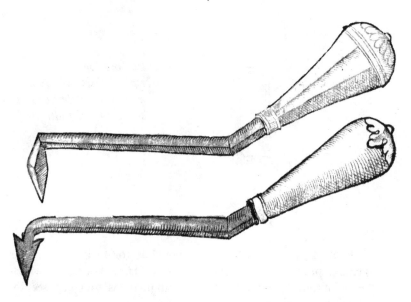

You will also be able to use the following trepan for the same purpose, which one uses principally on the cranium to separate the first table.

Exfoliative trepan with a small peg to hold it in the handle.

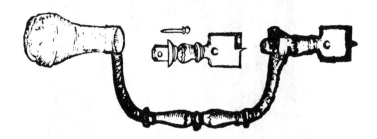

Especially you will be able to use the perforative trepan, of which you have the illustration here below, in piercing the carious bone in several parts of the caries and in going deeper until there comes out of it something like a bloody humidity, and this to give air and transpiration in order also that the virtue of the remedies can better consume the excessive moisture.

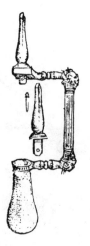

Perforative trepan with two points in triangle, and the little peg to serve to enhandle it.

Another trepan for the same use, but for making a greater opening, proper for the greatly carious large bones, of which the points are quadrangular or hexangular, as you can see by this following figure:

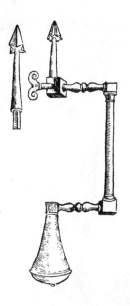

Trepan, whose points are quadrangular and hexangular.

Further, if the caries is very deep and the bone is solid (as is made often by alteration of the exterior air), then it is necessary to cut the diseased bones with the instruments which you see here, with which you will take away the corruption, striking thereon with a mallet, which should be of lead, in order to stun the part less. Then you will remove the fragments and splinters with small pincers which you see in this figure:

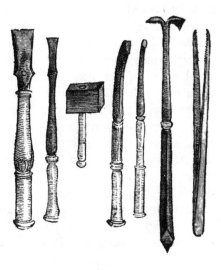

And if the caries is in a finger and there is no means of curing it, it will be necessary to use incisive tenacula, as you see by the following figure:

Incisive tenacula proper for cutting fingers.

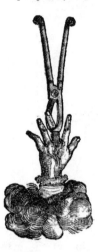

The sign for recognizing that one has removed the caries is when the bone above this is found more solid and when also one sees natural blood issue forth.

On actual and potential cauteries. Chapter 6.

And if these abovesaid instruments could not be used because of too great corruption, it would be best to use actual or potential cauteries. Of these I prize most the actual, because in strengthening the part they consume and dry the excessive fluids in the substance of the bone (which are the principal cause of the caries), which the potential cannot do as surely. Still, we are often constrained to use these because the patients often abhor the fire and the burning iron.

The potential are such as aqua fortis, water of copperas, hot oil, melted and boiling sulphur, and others similar. In the application of these, it is required that the surgeon exercise great discretion and ability, for there is danger that by default of industry and dexterity he may touch with these some part of the healthy flesh, which would be the cause of exciting great pains and inflammation (a thing greatly to be feared).

112

Greng, Penelope

As for the actual, they are made in so many sorts that the recital of them would be too long because of the diversity of the forms, which cannot be limited and even less written, because it is necessary to diversify them according to the extent of the lesion and shape of the carious bones. However, I shall present here some illustrations of those which are now most used for the said caries, of which some are knife-like, the others pointed, others olive-like, and of other shapes.

Different types of actual cauteries, which you will be able to use at your convenience.

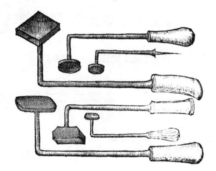

Other cauteries.

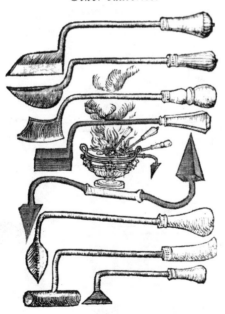

Other cauteries.

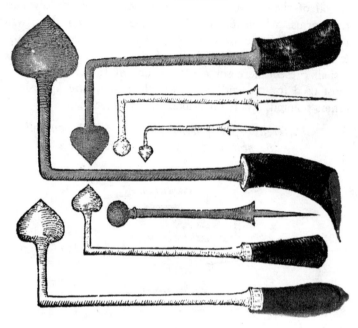

Other cauteries.

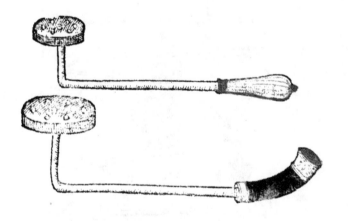

114

Other cauteries.

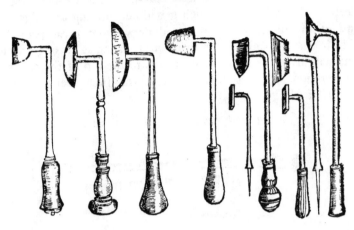

Other cauteries.

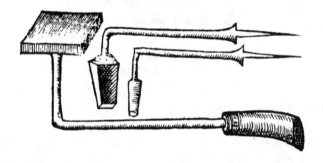

This following is proper for the nodes of smallpox which are on the cranium, when one wishes to remove the flesh which covers the bone. For this reason, it is hollowed and trenchant, of triangular and quadrangular shape, and separated into three to use them at your convenience.

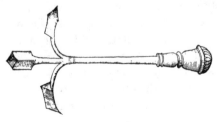

Those which follow will be useful if the carious bone is deep, so that one cannot touch it without burning the edges and lips of the ulcer, which is not done without great pain. For this, it is surer and gentler to use iron cannulae through which one will make the actual cautery pass to the top of the caries, in the fashion which follows, without the flesh feeling notable action of fire.

Actual cauteries with cannulae.

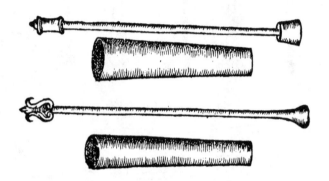

On the ill which comes from actual cauteries unduly applied. Chapter 7.

I must note here for you that if the cauteries are badly applied, that is to say too often, or if they are left on the bone too long, there follows great misfortune, for by their excessive warmth and dryness not only is the excessive moisture of the carious bone consumed, but also the substantial humor, which is to produce the separation of the caries and induce flesh and covering between the carious bone and the healthy which remains above. Wherefore the application of the cauteries will be made as long as the surgeon will see to be necessary and according to the length and depth of the caries, holding them on it until one sees some discharge in no way frothy come out through the porosities of the carious bone. Doing this, one will aid nature to exfoliate, separate, and cast out the corrupted bone. I wish indeed to warn you here of what you are to observe carefully in cauterizing caries of the bones, namely, if they are deep, as in the thigh, and other very fleshy parts. That is, that before the application of the cauteries you must well fortify and cover the parts around the wound or ulcer because the blood or humor contained in the wound, to which one gives an outlet, being warmed and altered by the fire, makes as much impression of burning on the flesh as it issues forth as would boiling oil.

On what remedies must be used after the application of actual cauteries. Chapter 8.

After the cauterization, in order to separate the bones and make the scales fall, one is to apply two or three times our oil heretofore named hot oil of puppies. And although it is very proper for this, I do not approve of one's applying it often because by its thin and humid oleaginous substance it could again injure the bone. For every rational surgeon is to take note (as I have said) of the nature of the parts for the treatment of these. Now, the bone is dryer than any other part of our body, wherefore thick, unctuous, and humid medicaments are contrary to it. Further, by the same reason the flesh which is near the bones, inasmuch as it is by nature dryer and approaching the temperament of the bones, requires also dryer medicaments. On the contrary, the farther it is from them, it needs less desiccative medicaments. Therefore, it behooves to use the oil with discretion. Sometimes, also, it will be necessary to agitate the bones gently in order to aid nature to separate them, without pulling them by violence, if one does not see them raised upward, and almost not to hold at all. And if the surgeon is indiscreet enough to pull the carious bone before nature has made a covering over that which is healthy, he will be the cause of a new alteration being made. For this, the surgeon is to note well this passage, which is of no little consequence. Furthermore, when nature has cast and exfoliated the carious bone, good care must be taken not to apply thereon any corrosive medicaments for fear of consuming the flesh that nature will have produced beneath, which being newly formed is soft as newly coagulated cheese, because the blood in it is recently hardened and thickened. However, it is necessary to beware of consuming it by acrid medicaments, for with time it hardens and forms itself in the manner of small pomegranate seeds, in which one sees the discharge reddish, smooth, even, glutinous, non-fetid, and then white.

This done, there will be made thereon applications of the capital powders of desiccative faculty without any sharpness, as those of root of iris of Florence, of washed aloes, and mastic, myrrh, barley flour, and the like. Then the wound must be lead to cicatrix, diversifying the remedies as the ill requires.

On the vulnerary potion. Chapter 9.

Now, if it came about that the separation of the carious bone, and consequently the consolidation of the wound, is not made as one desires and hopes, as much for the malignity of the air as from the cacochymia of the body, and also from the age of the caries, a vulnerary potion must be prescribed for the patient, which I have often done with fortunate outcome because nature aided by such a potion does admirable things.

℞ of sanicle, of bugle, of mouse-ear, of Alexandrine laurel, of herb bennett, of selfheal, of dandelion, of tips of bramble, of greater comfrey and of bruisewort, of quinquenerviae, of betony, of tips of hemp, of agrimony, of verbena, of osmund, of madder, of ground ivy, of strawberry plant, of bugloss, of gentian, of rupturewort, of omnium capillarium recentium, of true germander, of catnip, of cinquefoil, of tansy, of herb Robert, of each m. ss, of cleaned raisins, of scraped licorice, of seed of hypericum, and of holy thistle, of each ℥ i, of the three cordial flowers of each p. ii. Let them be cooked thoroughly in ordinary water; then at the end add of white wine and of rose honey, of cinnamon, as much as suffices, let decoction be made, which one will pass through the wine cloth, and one ounce and a half of it will be given to the patient in the morning two hours before eating.

As you will note here, if one does not find all the above herbs, one may content oneself with a part. Also, you are to understand that the ingredients of the above potion are to be diminished or increased as you will see to be necessary to the habits of the patient. I can assure you that I have seen by experience marvelous effects of this potion on old ulcers, malignant ulcers, and fistulas, which I could show by good reason. For as our body and our spirits are well if the nourishment we use is good and worthwhile, in the same way we are in trouble if the said nourishment is bad. Now, it is certain that he who has any ulcer, fistula, or arthritic passion, as soon as he becomes immoderate in his eating or drinking, as if he eats very salty viands, spices, garlics, or onions, strong wine, and without water, and other harmful things, at once feels pain and inflammation in his joints or in his ulcer, and likewise change of discharge from his ulcer. Whence I conclude that when you order the use of this potion, which has the faculty of purifying the sanguinary mass as much by urines and sweats as by vapors and impalpable perspiration, it will aid greatly in the cure of the said ulcers and fistulas, which we see by ordinary experience.

The surface of the bone does not fall alone, rather, the whole bone. Chapter 10.

To return to our purpose, it must be noted that not only does the surface of the bone not fall alone, but also a whole bone. This is shown by Hippocrates when he says the bone of the cranium, being wounded, separates from the healthy more or less according to the intensity of the blow; in addition, experience shows it, not only in this bone but in all the others. In this place I shall relate what I did in Piedmont where I was surgeon to my late Lord Marshal de Montjean* (who was then lieutenant for the King); I treated a lackey of the Seigneur de Goulaines who was wounded by a sword blow in the parietal bone of the left side, not penetrating as far as the second table. Some days after his wound was almost consolidated and cured there arrived at Turin a company of soldiers from his land of Gascony, with whom one morning he ate fried tripes, seasoned with plenty of onions and spices, which he did not do without drinking a great deal of wine, and good wine, to the point of remaining dead drunk. As a result, a day or two afterward he fell into a continued fever, lost his speech and his senses, and there developed a great swelling in his whole head and in his face, his eyes red and inflamed, issuing out of his head. Seeing this, I called several physicians and surgeons to advise on what could be necessary to save his life. We were all of the opinion of bleeding, clysterizing, cupping-glassing him, and of making

---

*René de Montjean (d. 1538), governor and lieutenant-general in Piedmont, 1537.

application of several remedies on his head, with frictions and bindings on his extremeties. Nevertheless, the whole side of the affected part abscessed several days later and, having made an opening, threw out a great quantity of discharge. I found the muscular skin separated from the cranium for the width of four fingers or about. Finally, both tables of the bone became altered, rotted, and black. To correct their corruption, I applied on the bone at certain intervals actual cauteries, this as much to correct the putrefaction as to make separation of what was altered and contrary to nature. About a month later, treating him I saw come out a certain quantity of worms from beneath the rotted bone by some holes which the caries had made in the bone, which caused me to hasten to pull and lift the said bone, which for a long time before had been shaking above the dura mater (where nature had formed flesh). I found three cavities large enough to put my thumb in, which were all full of moving worms, and each one in its place about as thick as the tag of a point, all having black heads. Now, the portion of the bone that nature had separated was as large as the palm of the hand, or more, such that on seeing it one could not comprehend that nature can cast out and separate such a quantity of the bone of the cranium without death. Still, he was finally cured beyond my hope and the hope of all those who had seen him. But after consolidation of his wound, the cicatrix remained greatly hollow (which is written by Hippocrates)* because of the destruction of the bone which is of original matter, which cannot be regenerated according to the first intention. And also because flesh cannot duly grow on a callus because it is as a foreign thing and unnatural, and especially because it is more solid and compact than the natural bone. Therefore, the blood cannot well sweat through it and consequently the flesh cannot be regenerated. As a result, when there is destruction of bone in some part of our body, the cicatrix always remains hollow. In the cranium where there is destruction of substance of the two tables, one sees it by the sense of sight, and one feels by the touch of the hand a pulsation made by the movement of the brain at the place of the cicatrix. Also, the place remains for a long space of time more infirm and painful. For this cause, I had made for the said lackey a bonnet of boiled leather in order

---

*Aphorisms, VI, 45: ulcera quaecumque.

to prevent external injuries, which he wore until the cicatrix was quite solid and the part fortified by some porus or callus made by the providence of nature, a thing worthy of great admiration. This will serve you as a conclusion for this discourse on caries.

End of the sixth book.

The Seventh Book

treats of gangrene and mortification and contains 21 chapters.

On Gangrenes and Mortifications

Book VII.

On gangrenes and mortifications. Chapter 1.

In all wounds and solutions of continuity (of which I have spoken here above) occur most often great and grievous complications as much for the inadvertence of the surgeon as by the faults which come from the patient, as well as from other external things or from the greatness of the malady. Principally among other complications come gangrene and mortification, which are of very great importance and peril of life if one does not remedy them diligently. For this reason, it has seemed to me good to write of gangrene and mortification, and this for two reasons. The one is that the said gangrene and mortification gave more evil to the surgeons, as well as to the patients, than the maladies in which they occur. As a result, it is necessary to give up the proper cure to obviate their furor and malignity. The other reason, which I have already declared heretofore, is a part of the causes of the said gangrene and mortification. However, I have wished to write of all of them more amply and of their cure, to the end that each one can have entire knowledge and cure them as appertains. I shall begin then with the definition. Then I shall declare to you the causes, their signs, prognosis, and consequently the cure that I shall give to be understood by example and familiar demonstration.

Definition of gangrene. Chapter 2.

Gangrene* is a disposition which tends to mortification of the wounded part which is not yet dead or wholly deprived of feeling but is dying little by little, so that if one does not soon give attention to it, it will completely mortify, indeed, as far as the bones. Then it is called by the Greeks, sphacelos or necrosis, by the Latins, syderatio, and estiomenos according to the Arabs and moderns, and by the vulgar, St. Anthony's or St. Marcel's fire.

On the general causes of gangrene. Chapter 3.

The first and general cause of gangrene is when, by the dissolution of the harmony or temperament of the four qualities, a part cannot receive the virtues or spirits which maintain it and preserve it in its state, that is, the natural spirit proceeding from the liver, carried by the veins to give it nourishment. Similarly, by the vital spirit, sent from the heart by the arteries to visit it. Also by the animal spirit sent from the brain by the nerves to give feeling and movement, which spirits received in the part preserve and restore the state and temperament of the part in its entirety. On the contrary, if by some hindrance the spirits are not communicated to that part, it must be corrupted and spoiled and its movement marred, which is the principal cause of gangrene and mortification, which also come from the other special and particular causes hereafter declared.

Galen, *Ad Glaucon*, II

On the particular causes of gangrenes.
Chapter 4.

The special causes are primary or antecedent. The primary or external are burns (by means of which come great inflammations) made actually or potentially; actually, as burns caused by fire, oil, water, cannon powder, or the like; potentially, by application of acrid medicaments, such as sublimate, vitriol, potential cauteries, or others. By freezing or great taking of colds by the air which surrounds us, or by undue applications of cold and stupefactive remedies, fractures, dislocations, great contusions or bruises, strong bindings, bites of venomous beasts or others not venomous, prickings of nerves or tendons, wounds made in the nervous parts, as in the joints or near these, or made in the plethoric and cacochymic bodies. Other wounds in which the vessels which bring life are completely or partly cut, whence to some follows what the Greeks call aneurysm, and other causes, which I leave for brevity.

On the antecedent causes of gangrene. Chapter 5.

The antecedent or internal and corporal causes are great flows of hot or cold humors, which fall on a part in greater quantities than it can alter, digest, and control by its faculties, so that such flows suffocate and extinguish the natural warmth and the spirits. For, because of the small and narrow space of the place, the arteries cannot have their natural movements, which are diastole, that is to say, dilatation, by which the exterior air is drawn in, and systole, which is contraction by which the fuliginous excrements are cast out through the pores or small passages of the said part. Furthermore, Galen says* that sometimes the inflammation begins in the bones, which is today quite manifest to us, not only simple inflammation but caries and corruption of the said bones, principally in the poxed and edematous or measled, whose flesh and skin appear healthy in some places and not corrupted, and beneath one finds the bones all putrefied, corroded, pierced, and full of worm holes, and even most often destruction of their proper substance, indeed in great quantity. This is done by a venomous matter whose quality cannot be expressed, and (as I have heretofore

---

*Des tumeurs contre nature

written) I can conclude that in such disposition there is divinity. Often times also, when the flesh of some part is ulcerated, there is developed a bad discharge, acrid and fetid, from which, if the bones are imbued, they are corrupted and mortify. This is seen happen often in filthy and malignant ulcers or others which have remained on any part for a long time. Also, Hippocrates testifies it*, saying that in all ulcers of a year or more old, the bone must separate and fall and deep and hollow scars remain. Similarly, the said gangrenes and mortifications occur by warm or cold venomous quality; warm, as one sees in carbuncles and pestiferous anthrax, that, in less than twenty-four hours, scab will be made and mortification in the affected part; cold, as one sees occur suddenly in a part without preceding pain or swelling or lividity or other signs of gangrene. De Vigo certifies he saw this happen to a noble woman of the city of Genoa. I remember also seeing similar done in this town of Paris to a man who was making good cheer during the day, not complaining of any pain. However, that night there came upon him gangrene and mortification in both legs without swelling or inflammation, but there was a color in certain places tending to lividity, blackness, and greenness. In some other places the color was almost natural. Still, there was no feeling, and when one pricked it with the point of the lancet or with a pin, no blood came out of it, and there was no warmth to the sense of touch. On the contrary, one felt rather a coldness.

Seeing this, I called council, by which it was deliberated and decreed that one would make many and deep incisions to attempt the cure. This I did, but from these incisions came out only a little very black, thick, and partially congealed blood. Many other remedies were attempted but, in spite of this, he rendered up his spirit to God with great delirium, having his face and whole body livid. I leave to be thought if the cause were not venomous. A similar case occurred to a certain person at Turin, the year one thousand five hundred and thirty-six, as I have heard by the recital made me by the late François Voste, a very learned surgeon, citizen of Turin. In this place, it will not be impertinent to declare and expose how gangrenes and mortifications are made by cold without

---

*Aphorisms, VI, 45

venomous quality, which I have only touched in a word in the external causes. Then, for greater clarity, I shall explain it to you.

Extreme cold, whether by the surrounding air or by application of cold and stupefactive repercussive remedies, makes a cold irregular temperature so great that the spirits are suffocated and extinguished. And when nature or the providence of the whole body sends other spirits to relieve the part, the said spirits, not finding the harmony well disposed for their reception, withdraw suddenly toward their origin, as though they were repulsed by the great cold of the part, hostile and completely contrary to nature. And therefore the said part, thus destitute of the said spirits, promptly mortifies. This is recognized manifestly in those who walk through snows and ices, for by the extreme cold they lose some of their members and quite often their lives, as presently we shall discuss.

I have good memory of having treated in Piedmont many soldiers who had passed the mountains in winter, some of whom by the extreme cold had lost their ears, others the half of an arm, others the virile member, others the toes of their feet, and some lost their lives; witness the chapel of the Trantiz situated on the mount of Sevy.

Also I remember that in the winter time a poor Breton stable servant, dwelling in Paris, after having drunk well went to lie down on a bed near which there was a half open window through which the cold entered and so altered one of his legs that on his awakening, thinking to get up, he could not stand. However, he was placed near the fire to which he brought his leg, thinking only that it was asleep, but he burned the sole of his foot the thickness of a finger without feeling anything because it was already more than half mortified by the cold. The next day, the said Breton was brought to the Hostel Dieu where he was visited by the surgeon and others, who concluded that it was necessary to cut and amputate the mortified leg, which was done. But, nevertheless, the mortification gained the upper parts so that within three days after the said Breton died with cold sweat, delirium, great eructations, and syncopes. Moreover, in the said time of winter, it was so very cold that the extremities of the noses of some patients bedded in the Hostel Dieu mortified without any putrefaction, and I amputated the said part from four of these, of whom two were cured; the others died. Since I have discussed amply all the causes of gangrene and mortification, I must proceed to the declaration of the signs of the said gangrene and mortification, which I shall distinguish according to their causes in order to give to young surgeons, not yet experienced, the entire knowledge of the said gangrene and mortification and of their causes.

On the signs of gangrenes. Chapter 6.

The signs of gangrenes made by phlegmonic inflammation are when the great pain and pulsation, which had preceded the said inflammations, are greatly diminished, and the reddish or vermilion color, which was previously in the part, is changed into pale, cyanotic color, somewhat tending to lividity. I mean here pulsatile pain, not that which is made by the movement of the arteries, but a jerking or stinging pulsation, which is made when by the combat between the two warmths (that is, natural and non-natural), several vapors arise from the humors and matters which tend to putrefaction in the inflamed parts. If the cold is cause of the gangrene and mortification, it will be easy to recognize. For (as each one knows), the great cold promptly makes in the part great poignant and cutting pain and shining redness, and soon after renders it livid and very cold and seemingly without movement and feeling, with horror or trembling, as if one had a beginning of quartan fever. If the cold continues longer than the warmth of the part can resist, gangrene will occur and, consequently, mortification (if one does not take care of it) and finally death. For, as Hippocrates says*, cold is contrary and hostile to the bones, teeth, nerves, to the brain, to the marrow of the back, generally to our life (which consists in warmth and humidity), because it makes spasms or convulsions and other movements against our will, disordered agitation of the whole body (which we call chills), and consequently by its great violence is often times the cause of our death.

As for gangrenes and mortifications made by strong bindings, fractures, dislocations and great contusions, you will recognize them easily by the lividity and color of the dead part, for because of the compression, the spirits cannot deliver to the

---

*Aphorisms, V, 18

part its natural color. The signs discussed in the gangrenes engendered by inflammation will be able to give you knowledge of the gangrenes made by bites, stings, aneurysms, wounds made in plethoric and cacochymic bodies, for by these causes is made too great flow and attraction of humors which hinder (as I have said) the air and ventilation of the part. As for the signs of gangrene and mortification coming from venom, there is no need for reciting them here as one can recognize and distinguish the complications which come from warm as well as cold venoms, for I have written of them heretofore in speaking of poisoned arrows, which place one can see.

On the prognosis of gangrenes. Chapter 7.

Then, after one has recognized gangrene and mortification by its signs and causes, it is necessary, before attempting anything of the cure, to consider what effect the disposition can have and predict and indicate it to the patients or their friends (which we call prognostication), as I shall tell you. Gangrene and mortification are of such great ferocity and malignity that if one does not remedy it promptly, the part easily and completely will die and will corrupt the near parts, because such corruption makes its way through the whole part as venom and corrodes it as does a fire kindled in dry wood, until finally the patients will die. And before they die, they all have a general cold sweat with delirium or reveries, syncopes or faintings, eructations and hiccups, because the vapors raised by the putrefaction and rotting are communicated and carried by the veins, arteries, and nerves to the noble parts. Your prognosis made, it is necessary to put the hand to the work, as I shall discuss now.

On the general cure of gangrene. Chapter 8.

In the treatment of gangrene, it is necessary to take the indications of the malady, for it is necessary to diversify the cure according to the essence or greatness of the ill, because some gangrenes and mortifications occupy a whole part, others only a portion. Some are deep, others superficial. Such diverse causes make the cure diversified. To all causes it is not fitting to apply the same remedy. Similarly, it is necessary to consider the temperament of the body and of the part. For some (as we have said heretofore) are of soft and delicate temperament, as women, young children, idle people living delicately, eunuchs, and others. These demand milder and less violent remedies than those who are of hard and robust habits or substance, as laborers, mariners, boatmen, hunters, porters, and other laboring people. Not only is it necessary to have this consideration of the body, but also of the wounded parts. For there is a difference in the muscular and fleshy parts, as arm or leg; or nervous, hard and solid parts, as vertebrae, joints, and others; also in the warm and humid parts, as are the shameful parts, the mouth, the womb, the anus, in which corruption and putrefaction come more promptly than in the other parts of our body. Therefore, according to the essence, temperament, and natural disposition of these parts and of the body, it is necessary to administer remedies and proceed to the cure.

And among the other remedies, it is necessary to order good regimen and manner of living on the six non-natural things, to obviate and oppose (as much as will be possible for us) the malady and its cause, if it is still present. If the habit of the body is plethoric or cacochymic, it is necessary to bleed or purge according to the counsel of the physician. And inasmuch as the vapors which rise from the gangrened part are communicated by the arteries to the heart and subsequently to the other noble parts, it is necessary to strengthen the heart so that it will not be infected by these malignant vapors by giving to drink theriac dissolved in water of small sorrel, or holy thistle, mithridate to eat and conserve of roses or bugloss, opiates and other cordial things which have been discussed above. One can also apply this poultice outside on the region of the heart in order always to strengthen:

℞ of waters of roses, of nenuphar, of each ℥ iiii, of squillitic vinegar ℥ i, of corals and of sandalwood, white and red, of red roses, of powder of risatarum and of spodium, of each ℥ i, of mithridate, of theriac, of each ℈ ii ss, of troches of camphor ℈ ii, of cordial flowers, pulverized, p. ii, of crocus ℈ i. Let all be dissolved together, let epithem be made, which is placed over the heart with scarlet cloth of sponge.

There briefly is the summary of the general things, and we must now come to the proper and specific cure of gangrenes.

On the specific cure of gangrene. Chapter 9.

The cure of gangrene made by flow of blood and other humors which suffocate the part, as one sees happen often in great inflammations, is to be made by evacuating and drying promptly the corrupted blood and humors which are arrested in the suffering part. This is to be done with many scarifications and incisions, large, medium, small, deep, and superficial according to need and necessity in order that the said part can ventilate and air itself and exhale the corrupted vapors. One makes incisions when the ill is great, deep, and near putrefaction, and scarifications when it begins to putrefy. For as great as the ill is, there is need of great and violent remedies. Therefore, if the said ill goes as far as the bones, it is necessary to divide the skin and the flesh with many deep incisions that you will be able to make with this razor proper and suitable for this:

Razor.

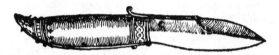

Still, you must take care not to touch the notable nerves and vessels if they are not wholly rotten and corrupted. For in this case it is necessary to make incision without regard for the said vessels. But if they are intact, the incisions are to be made between the vessels without touching them. If the gangrene is minor, there is need of scarifications only.

After the scarifications and incisions are made, it is necessary to let a great deal of blood flow in order to evacuate the conjoined matter, discharge, and dry the part. Then apply remedies which have the faculty of taking away the putrefaction by their warming, desiccative, resolvent, detersive, and aperitive virtues, and of penetrating deeply in order to consume the virulent and corrupted matter which is arrested and fixed in the gangrened part. And for this purpose, you will make ablution with lye made of ashes of fig tree or of oak, in which lupines have been boiled until they are perfectly cooked. Or to have remedies more easy to come by, it is necessary to take salted water, in which aloes and Egýptiac have been boiled, adding at the end some brandy.

Another:

℞ of best vinegar lb. i, of rose honey ℥ iiii, of acetous syrup ℥ iii, of common salt ℥ v. Let them boil together, add of brandy lb. ss. With these ablutions it is necessary to wash the parts several times, for they are of great efficacy in gangrenes. These said ablutions made, you will apply Egyptiac on compresses, for it is the most excellent and first in dignity among the remedies suitable to putrefactions because it separates the rotten from the scab-forming healthy flesh; thus it is not necessary to await the fall of the rottenness, but rather to cut it and take away what is corrupted with razor or scissors. Then apply again the said Egyptiac as many times as needed. This you will recognize by the color of the flesh, by the stinking and sensitivity of the subjacent parts. The description of the said Egyptiac (from which I have always known great effects in these cases) is such:

℞ of flowers of copper, of rock alum, of common honey, of each ℥ iii, of sharpest vinegar ℥ v, of common salt ℥ i, of Roman vitriol ℥ ss, of pulverized sublimate ℈ ii. Let them all boil together on the fire; let ointment be made. If there is need, one will make it less strong. With the application of the said Egyptiac, it is necessary to put on the whole affected part this cataplasm, which prevents and prohibits putrefaction, resolves, cleanses, dries, and quiets the pain.

℞ of flour of beans, of barley, of bitter vetch, of lentils, of lupines, of each lb. ss, of common salt and of rose honey, of each ℥ iiii, of juice of absinthe, of horehound, of each ℥ ii ss, of aloes, of mastic, of myrrh, and of brandy of each ℥ ii, of simple oxymel as much as suffices. Let soft cataplasm be made according to the art.

The said remedies consume, resolve, and cleanse the virulent discharge and putrid matter and, by their great dryness and tenuity of essence penetrating to the depth, prevent the putrefaction, quiet the pain, and strengthen the part, which is most necessary in such case. One is also to apply above the ill such or a similar defensive to obviate and repress the descent of the humors and to take care that the rotten vapors raised from the putrefaction do not rise to the heart or to the superior and noble parts.

℥ of rose oil, of myrtle, of each ℥ four, of juice of plantain, of nightshade, of leek, of each ℥ two, whites of eggs five in number, of Armenian bole, of sealed earth finely pulverized, of each ℥ one, of oxycrate as much as suffices; mix for the use said.

One can also make others having similar virtue, but it must be noted that these remedies must be renewed often. Now, if the ill is so great that it does not wish to yield to the aforesaid remedies, it is necessary to come to others more vehement and violent, which are cauteries. After the application of these Galen in the second *To Glaucon* commands that juice of leeks with crushed and dissolved salt be put on because such remedy penetrates and dries strongly and by this means prevents putrefaction. Further, if the said cauteries do not profit, there is need to come to the extreme, which is to amputate the part, according to the saying of Hippocrates*: In extreme maladies, extreme and last remedies are fitting. Still, one is not to do this unless one first has certain knowledge whether the part is totally dead. For it is not a small case to cut off a member, if it is not more than necessary. Therefore, I shall give you entire and infallible knowledge of the complete mortifications and gangrenes by the signs put hereafter.

On the signs of complete mortifications. Chapter 10.

If one recognizes in the affected part blackness and coldness coming from the extinction of the natural flesh, not from the surrounding air; great softness, which if one compresses it cannot raise itself up again, rather there remains there a cavity or fossa; separation of the skin from the subjacent flesh; great stinking, as from a corpse (principally if the said gangrene is an ulcer), the smell of which is so sharp and strong that it is intolerable and abominable to all persons; and there comes out of it a viscid liquid of black and greenish color; principally total privation of feeling and movement, whether one pulls, strikes, presses, burns, cuts, touches, or pricks, certainly you can conclude a perfect mortification or gangrene.

Still it is necessary to explore the loss of feeling with good judgment. For I know that many have been deceived trusting in a feeling that the patients say they have if one pricks, presses, or therewise touches, which is totally false and deceptive. For it comes only from a great apprehension of the extreme pain which previously was in the part, and principally by the

---

Aphorisms, I, 6

continuity and consent that the dead parts still have with the live. As, for a familiar example, we see that if one pulls our shirt or other garment adhering to our body, we say we feel it although the garment is insensitive and only contiguous to our body. Of this false feeling you will have manifest argument after the amputation of the mortified parts. For the patients, long after the amputation is made, say they still feel pain in the dead and amputated parts. Of this they complain strongly, a thing worthy of wonder, and almost incredible to people who have not experienced this. Therefore, it is necessary to take care that such feeling not delay us in performing the duty of perfect cure, as I have sometimes seen a member cut two or three times for having stopped at a false and uncertain feeling. Then, after having recognized that the part is truly dead, it is necessary promptly and without delay, however small it may be, to cut and amputate it, for the contagion and corruption ravishes and gains without cease the neighboring healthy and live parts. This remedy is miserable and worthy of compassion, to the patient as well as to the surgeon, but it is the only and last refuge, which one must still prefer to death, which will follow if one seeks other means than section of the mortified part.

On the place where it is necessary to begin the amputation. Chapter 11.

It does not suffice, however, to recognize that it is necessary to amputate the mortified part, but it is necessary to know the place where one is to make and begin the amputation. In that lies the judgment and prudence of the surgeon. The art commands that one begin at the healthy part, but I shall declare this to you easily. Let us put down, for example, that someone has a gangrene in his foot as far as the malleoli or ankle. In such case, it is necessary to consider well where you are to make the amputation, for according to the art, it is necessary to keep the human body entire as much as is possible. Therefore, you are to take away the least that you can of the healthy part. Nevertheless, it is necessary to have consideration of the action and adornment of the part, which will make it advisable to cut the leg at five fingers or about near the knee, because the amputation made in this place, the part will afterward be better able to do its action, which will be to walk with a wooden leg. For if one should cut only a little above the lesion, the patient would be in difficulty of carrying three legs, where he will carry only two. I know that Captain François Le Clerc, being on a ship, had a cannon shot which carried away his foot a little above the ankle, of which wound he was cured. But some time afterward, seeing that his leg hurt him, he had it cut as far as five fingers near the knee. Now he finds he walks better than he did before. In the arm, it is necessary to do the contrary, which is to take away the least that one can of the healthy part because of the difference in the actions of the arm and of the leg. I have discussed heretofore how one will be able to recognize the necessity of section and the place of it. It is now necessary to show the means of proceeding and exercising the said section.

On the means of proceeding to the section of the member.
Chapter 12.

In the first place, you will strengthen the force and strength of the patient, if there is need, by proper foods of easy digestion and full of spirits, as soft eggs, roast steeped in good wine, or others similar. Then place the patient in the proper position and pull the muscles upward toward the healthy part and make an extremely tight ligature a little above the place that you will wish to amputate with a strong delicate band, and of flat shape, like those with which women bind their hair. This ligature serves for three things; the first is that with the aid of the assistant it holds the skin and muscles raised upward, in order that after the amputation they may recover the ends of the bones which have been cut, and after the healing, the scar formed, the skin and muscles serve as a cushion to the said extremities of the bones. Thus, the part will be able to remain stronger and less painful upon pressure. Along with that, the healing is shorter, for the more flesh one leaves on the bones, the sooner they are covered. The second is that it prohibits hemorrhaging or flow of blood because it presses the veins and arteries. The third is that it makes dull and greatly takes away feeling from the part, because it impedes by its great compression the animal spirit which gives feeling to the part by the nerves. Then, after the strong ligature is thus made, it is necessary promptly to cut all the muscles and other parts as far as the bone with a well-cutting razor or knife curved as that following:

Knife curved for cutting the members.

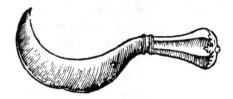

Now, it is necessary for you to note here that there is between the bones portions of some muscles which you will not be able to cut well with the said razor or knife; however, you will cut them with such an instrument made in the manner of a curved lancet. I warn you of this, for if you leave anything other than the bone to cut with the saw, certainly in sawing you will cause great pain to the patient, because the saw can only with great difficulty cut soft things such as flesh, tendons, and membranes as it does the hard and solid bones.

Curved lancet.

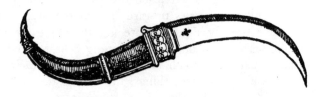

After having entirely cut all the parts to the bones, it is necessary to saw them properly with such a saw:

Saw.

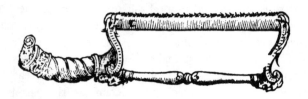

On the means of arresting the flow of blood when the member is cut. Chapter 13.

When the amputation of the member is made, it is necessary that some quantity of blood flow, in order that fewer complications occur to the relieved part, and this according to the strength and plethora of the sick person. This Hippocrates teaches us*, saying that there is need for recent ulcers to let some quantity of blood flow, except the stomach, because the part will be less molested by inflammation and consequently the ulcer will cure sooner. He says likewise that it is good to make old ulcers bleed often, in order that by this means the part which can not assimilate the blood which is sent to it for its nourishment by reason of its debility is discharged and rendered stronger. The blood having flowed in sufficient quantity (always taking indication of the strength of the sick person), it is necessary to ligature promptly the large veins and arteries so firmly that they do not flow any more. This will be done by taking the above vessels with such an instrument named crow's beak.

Crow's beak proper for drawing the vessels to bind them.

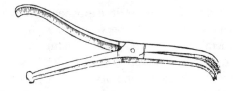

With this instrument, it is necessary to pinch the vessels, pulling them and drawing them out of the flesh, into which they are withdrawn and hidden, as do all other parts, always toward their origin. Doing this you need not be too careful of pinching only the vessels because there is no danger of taking with them some portion of the flesh of the muscles or other parts, for from this cannot come any complication. Rather with this, the union of the vessels will be made better and more surely than if there were only the body of the vessels included in the ligature. Thus drawn, they are to be well tied with good thread which is doubled.

---

*On ulcers

137

*How it is necessary to proceed with the treatment of
an amputated member, the flow of blood arrested.
Chapter 14.*

This done, you will untie the first ligature that you had
made above the place of the cut. Then promptly you will make
four stitches with a needle in cross form in the lips of the wound,
deepening the said stitches one finger in the flesh in order that
they hold more firmly. By this means, you will bring the
parts of the cut muscles back over the bone in order that it
be better and more quickly covered and less touched by the
surrounding air, in order that the said flesh serve it as a
cushion after the consolidation. Now, you are to note that it is
not necessary to press the stitches so close that you strive to
bring the lips of the wound together, which also you will not
be able to do. Rather, it will suffice to press them partially
together in order to bring the skin and subjacent flesh back
to the position and parallel length in which they were before
the retraction which was made after and during the amputation.

*What must be done if there occurs flow of blood because
one of the abovesaid vessels becomes untied. Chapter 15.*

These things thus done, if it happened afterward that any
one of the said vessels should become untied, it is necessary to
rebind the member with your first ligature as has been said
heretofore or, in place of doing this (which I advise more and
which is very much easier and less painful), that an assistant
take the member in his two hands, pressing strongly with his
fingers on the place of the path of the said vessels, for by
doing this he will prevent the flow of blood. Meanwhile, you
will take a needle four inches long or about, squared and sharp,
threaded with good thread doubled three or four times, with
which you will bind the vessels in the following fashion, for then
the crow's beak could not serve you. You will pass the said
needle through the outside of the wound, at a half finger or
more, beside the said vessel, across the wound, near the orifice
of the vessel. Then you will pass it again under the vessel, compressing it with your thread, and you will make your needle
come out in the exterior part on the other side of the vessel,
leaving between the two paths of the needle only the space of
a finger. Then you will tie your thread rather tightly over

a small compress of linen doubled two or three times, of the thickness of a finger, which will guard against the knot's entering the flesh and will stop it securely. The ligature retracts entirely within the mouth and orifice of the vein or artery, with which, also concealed and covered by the adjacent fleshy parts, the orifice easily is reknit. I can assure you that after such an operation one never sees a drop of blood come out of the vessels thus tied. And it is not necessary to belabor oneself to use the above means of arresting the blood in the small vessels because it will easily be suppressed by the astringents that we shall prescribe for you hereafter.

You may find this manner of practicing rather obscure and difficult to understand, but you must consider that it is a very difficult thing to put manual surgery clearly and entirely in writing, for it is rather to be learned by imagination and by seeing good and experienced masters perform, if you have the means or, indeed, to try it on dead bodies, as I have done many times.

On emplastic medicaments. Chapter 16.

Now we shall tell the remedies which it behooves to use after the amputation of the member, which are the adhesives greatly proper to recent wounds, as are these:

℞ of Armenian bole ℥ iiii, of volatile flour ℥ iii, of pitch, of resin ℥ ii. Let all be pulverized very finely, and mixed together, let powder be made; with which the wound will be completely powdered, then garnished above with dry scraped lint. Afterward one will apply on top this repellant:

℞ of whites of eggs, in number vi, of Armenian bole, of dragon's blood, of gypsum, of sealed earth, of aloes, of mastic, of burnt galls, of each ℥ ii. Let them be pulverized very finely and stirred well, adding rose oil and myrtle, of each ℥ i. Let defensive be made in the form of honey.

This ointment is to be applied on the part, and a little higher, with stupes steeped in oxycrate. Thus, if you have cut the leg it is necessary to apply your ointment four fingers or more above the knee. This remedy is not only repellent but also strengthens the part, prevents discharge, calms the flow of blood, quiets the pain, and prevents fever. Moreover, it is necessary to steep in oxycrate the compresses and bandages, then place the member in mid-position on cushions and pillows full of oat straw, deer hair, or of bran. The above dressing is not to be renewed without great necessity, that is, four days after in winter, and less in summer, according as you see there is need.

I confess here freely and with great regret that I have heretofore practiced quite otherwise, after the amputation of arms and legs was made, than I am writing at this hour. But what? I had seen thus done by those who were called for such practices, in which immediately after the member was extirpated they used many cauteries, actual as well as potential, to prevent the flow of blood, a thing very horrible and cruel even to relate, for that caused an extreme pain to the patients considering that such wounds recently made are very sensitive. By reason of this sensitivity if one applied caustic things on and against the nervous parts, suddenly their action and impression is communicated to the internal parts, whence arise very great and pernicious complications and most often death. Truly, one never saw of six thus cruelly treated, two escape. Even they were ill for a long time, with difficulty were the wounds thus burned brought to consolidation, because such a burning made the pains so vehement that the sick ones fell into fever, spasm, and other mortal complications. Along with this, most often when the scab separated, there arose a new flow of blood so that it was necessary again to staunch it with actual and potential cauteries, which repeated consumed a great quantity of flesh and other nervous parts. As a result of this wasting away, the bones remained afterward naked and uncovered. For many this has rendered cicatrization impossible; all the rest of their lives they kept an ulcer in the place of the cut member, which took from them the means of being able to make use of a member made artificially. Wherefore I counsel the young surgeon to leave such cruelty and inhumanity in order rather to follow this my lesson of practicing, of which it has pleased God to advise me, without my ever having seen it done by anyone, heard it said, or read it, except in Galen in the fifth book of his *Method*, where he writes that it is necessary to tie the vessels toward their roots, which are the liver and the heart, in order to staunch the great flow of blood.

Now, having many times used this manner of sewing the veins and arteries in recent wounds in which a hemorrhaging took place, I have thought that as much could well be done in the extirpation of a member. I conferred on this with Estienne de la Riviere, surgeon ordinary of the King, and François Rasse, both surgeons at Paris, and having declared to them my opinion, they were of the advice that we should make the test of it on the first sick person who should offer himself, although we should have the cauteries all ready to use them in case of failure of the ligature. This I have practiced in the case of many, with very good results, again lately a few days ago on the person of a postilion, the servant of Brusquet, named Pirou Garbier, whose right leg was cut off, four fingers below the knee. for an eating away which had come to him because of a fracture.

I counsel the young surgeon to abandon this miserable manner of burning and butchering, admonishing him not to say any more, "I have seen it in the book of the ancient practitioners, I have seen it done by my old fathers and masters, following whose practice I can in no way fail." This I grant you if you wish to listen to your good master Galen in the book referred to above, and those like him, but if you wish to stop at your father and your masters in order to have prescriptioners of time and license of ill-doing, wishing always to persevere in it, such as one does to a certain degree ordinarily in all things, you will render account of it before GOD and not before your father or your good practitioner masters, who treat men in so cruel a fashion.

The manner of pursuing the treatment of the amputed member. Chapter 18.

Now, to take up again our first point and to finish thoroughly the cure begun by means of remedies proper and suitable to our ulcers, it is necessary first to note that before removing the ligatures with which the vessels have been bound it is important that the agglutination of these be made and that they be covered with flesh for fear of a new flow of blood.

This will be done by applying thereon some cold, astringent, and adhesive remedies such as the powder which follows:

℞ of powder of Armenian bole, of flour of barley, of pitch, of resin, of gypsum, of each ℥ iiii, of aloes, of nuts of cypress, of rind of pomegranate, of each ℥ i. Let all be incorporated together; let fine powder be made with which the whole ulcer will be sprinkled and powdered for the space of three or four days, then afterward one will use it only on the place of the vessels which have been bound and it will again be continued for the space of eight or ten days, in order that one may be well assured that the vessels are stopped and covered with flesh, but on the rest of the ulcer a digestive will be applied and continued until it has turned to suppuration. For then one will quit the digestive to take cleansing medicaments as those which follow:

℞ of Venice turpentine washed in brandy ℥ vi, of rose honey strained ℥ iii, of juice of plantain, of celery, and of lesser centaury, of each ℥ ii. Let all boil together as far as the consumption of juices, let them be removed from the fire, adding flour of barley and beans, of each ℥ i, of Galen's theriac ℥ ss, of aloes, of myrrh, of birthwort, of each ℈ iii, of crocus ℈ i. Let cleanser be made.

Now, it is so that a long time after the amputation, the patients think they still have in its entirety the member which has been amputated from them (as I have said). This happens to them, as it seems to me, because the nerves withdraw toward their origin and in withdrawing make great pain, almost similar to the retractions which are made in spasms. To remedy this, it is necessary to rub the nape of the neck and the whole affected part with the liniment which follows, and which is of great efficacy against spasm, paralysis, stupor, contortions, distentions, and other affections, principally of the nervous parts, arising from cold causes.

℞ of sage, of chamepitheos, of marjoram, of rosemary, of mint, of rue, of lavender, of each m. i, of flowers of camomile, of melilot, of tips of dill and of hypericum, of each p ii, of bays of laurel and of juniper, of each ℥ ii, of root of pellitory ℈ ii, of mastic, of sweet gum, of laserwort, of each ℥ i ss, of Venice turpentine lb. i, of oil of earthworms, of dill, and of puppies, of each ℥ vi, of oil of turpentine ℥ iii, of human fat ℥ ii, of crocus ℈ i, of fragrant white wine lb. i, of wax as much as suffices. Let the things to be crushed be crushed; let the things to be pulverized be pulverized; then let all be soaked in wine over night, afterward let them be cooked with the oils and the fat aforesaid in a double vase. Let liniment be made according to the art; at the end add of brandy ℥ iii.

Further, in treating this wound, it is fitting to procure the separation of the extremities of the bones which the saw and the air have touched. This the surgeon will do by the application of actual cauteries on the said bones, in the application of which he is to take good care not to touch the sensitive parts in any way but to use them discreetly as I have described heretofore. In doing this, you will note that the bones are not to be pulled by violence but by shaking them little by little. From this, nevertheless, you are to hope for the separation from thirty days or more after the amputation. This done, you will use remedies proper to consume the spongy and excess flesh, as do burnt vitriol, powder of mercury, and others, among which alum cooked and pulverized is very convenient if one applies it alone or with other cleansers. You will be able to use these remedies until the entire cure and cicatrization of the ulcers and change them as you shall see that there is need of it.

The means of accommodating artificial hands, arms, and legs in the place of the extirpated members. Chapter 19.

And although it be a very inhuman thing to extirpate a member thus, nevertheless we must place the life of the whole body ahead of the loss of a part of it, especially of the members that one can extirpate with hope of cure. What is more, usage has given us the means of imitating nature and supplying the default of the members lost, as you will see in the artificial members which we will describe hereafter.

Description of the figure of the wooden leg for the poor.

aa. Represents the trunk of the leg.
bb. The two forks for inserting the thigh, the shortest of which is to be put inside the leg.
cc. Shows you the small cushion which is put to support the leg softly on the roundness of the trunk.
dd. Are the thongs with buckles crossing the forks of the thigh in two spots to press it and to hold it between these.

By e. is marked for you the thigh in order to teach you the true position of it on the said wooden leg.

Wooden leg for the poor.

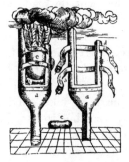

The figures and portraits of the arms and legs which follow represent the voluntary movements as closely as possible. For the flexion and extension can be made by arms and legs artificially made according to those portraits, which I have by great begging obtained from one named Le Petit Lorrain, locksmith residing at Paris, a man of good mind, with the names and explanation of each part of the said portraits made in proper terms and words of the artisan, in order that each locksmith, clock maker, or other worker handling iron can understand them and make artificial and similar arms and legs which serve not only for the action of the amputated parts, but also for the beauty and ornament of these, as one can recognize and see by the following figures:

Artificial leg.

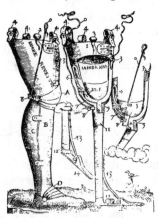

Description of the wooden leg.

0. The bond by which one pulls the ring of the catch in order to fold the leg.
1. The thigh guard with screws, and the holes of the screws to enlarge or restrict on the thigh, which will be within.
2. The pommel to place and support the hand and to turn oneself.
3. The little ring which is front of the thigh, to direct and guide the leg where one wishes.
4. The two buckles in front, and that behind, to hold and attach to the body of the doublet.
5. The little socket at the bottom, within which the thigh is put up to two fingers near the end, serving also to make the beauty and form of the leg.
6. The spring, to make the catch move which makes the leg firm.
7. The catch which holds the stick of the leg straight and firm, for fear that it may turn back.
8. The ring to which is attached a cord to pull the catch, in order that the stick can fold, when one sits and when one is on horseback.
9. The hinge to make the leg play and move, put in front of the knee.
10. A little stock or stop to keep the catch from passing beyond the thigh guard, for if it passed beyond, the spring would break and the man would fall.
11. The iron band in which the stick is inserted.
12. The other band at the end of the stick, which carries the hinge to make the foot move.
13. A spring to make the foot recover and throw it back into its place.
14. The stop which serves the spring for throwing the foot down again.

Dressed Leg.

A. Plates for the beauty of the leg.
B. The greave for the beauty and form of the leg.
C. The thickness to finish the form of the leg.
D. Plates for forming the ankle.

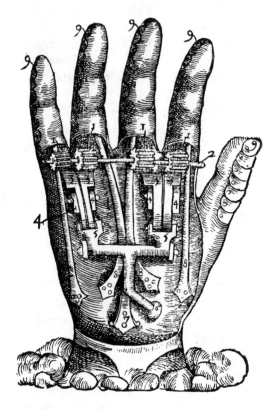

Description of iron hand.

1. Gears serving each finger, which are of the same piece as the fingers, added and assembled in the back of the hand.
2. Iron rod which passes through the middle of the said gears, on which they turn.
3. Catches to hold each finger firm.
4. Stocks or stops of the catches, in the middle of which are pegs to stop the catches.
5. The large catch to open the four small catches, which hold the fingers closed.
6. The button of the tail of the large catch, which, if pushed, the hand will open.
7. The spring which is below the large catch, serving to make it return to its place and hold the hand closed.

8. The springs of each finger, which bring back and make the fingers open of themselves when they are closed.
9. The plates of the fingers.

The following figure shows you the outside of the hand and the means of attaching it to the arm and to the sleeve of the doublet.

Description of the iron arm put hereafter.

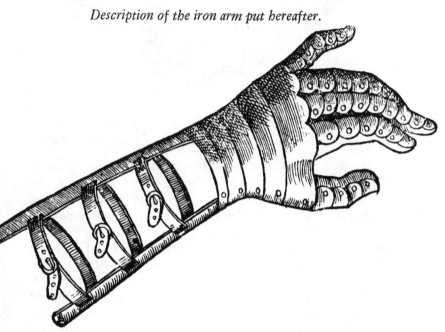

1. The iron bracelet for the form of the arm.
2. The tree put inside the large spring to extend it.
3. The large spring which is in the elbow, which is to be of tempered steel and three feet or more in length.
4. The ratchet.
5. The catch.
6. The spring which presses on the catch and stops the teeth of the ratchet.
7. The screw to fasten the spring.
8. The curve of the forearm which is above the elbow.
9. The trunk of the gauntlet made to bend with the barrel of the forearm which is to the hand, which serve to make the

hand prone and supine, that is, prone toward the earth and supine toward the sky.

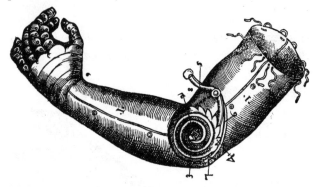

Memorable story of a mortification which happened to a soldier whose arm was cut at the elbow joint. Chapter 20.

I consider that I have rather amply discussed the means of treatment of gangrene and sphacelation, still, in order that you may better understand what I have said, I shall give you a recital (as an example) of a cure that I made at Turin in the service of my lord the Marshal de Montjean. A poor soldier received an arquebus shot in his left arm near the carpus and joint of the hand. As a result of this, the bullet had lacerated and broken many bones, tendons, and other nervous parts, whence arose gangrene, then an eating away as far as the joint of the elbow and the arm. From the elbow to the shoulder there was gangrene, and in the half of the thorax there was great inflammation and, indeed, notable evidence of gangrene. As a result of this, the patient had great eructations, syncopes, uneasiness, and other bad complications, announcing death. Because of this, the soldier was abandoned by several surgeons, and then I was stimulated by some of his friends to visit him, which I did, and after having recognized the mortification, I took the boldness according to the command of our art to amputate his arm at the joint of the elbow.

In the first place, I bound his arm tightly above the elbow for the reasons already given. This done, I cut off his arm without a saw, because the mortification was not beyond the joint of the elbow; and there I began the amputation, incising the ligaments which join the bones. The incision made, notwithstanding the ligature, there occurred a great flow of blood because of the vessels which are in this part. This I let flow sufficiently to discharge, relieve, and ventilate the part and also to dry the gangrene which was in the arm already tending to mortification. Then I stopped the blood with actual cauteries, not having at that time any other method or fashion of doing. This done, I untied the ligature gently, and afterward I made on the gangrene many large and deep incisions, avoiding the internal part of the arm because of the great veins, arteries, and multitude of nerves which are there. And moreover, I cauterized some of the incisions, as much to stop the blood as to dry and consume any virulent matter imbued in the part. Then I applied remedies, heretofore written, on the part, and on the inflammation of the thorax a great quantity of astringents and repellents; likewise, poultices over the heart and other cordial things that I gave him. These remedies I continued until the eructations and other complications which had occurred as a result of the vapors raised from the rottenness and communicated to the heart by the arteries were quieted and appeased.

Now I can not omit relating, to put one on his guard, that two weeks afterward there occurred to the poor soldier a spasm, which I had before prognosticated because of the cold and because he was badly couched in an attic where he not only had little covering but also was exposed to all the winds, without fire and other things necessary to human life. Seeing him in such spasm and contraction of the extremities, his teeth clenched, his lips and all his face twisted and pulled back as if he wanted to smile the *risus sardonicus*, which are manifest signs of convulsion, I was moved by pity. Desiring to do the due of my art, not being able to do any other thing for him then, I had him put in a stable in which was a large number of cattle and a great quantity of manure. Then I found means of having fire in two warmers near, while I rubbed the nape of his neck, arms and legs, avoiding the pectoral parts, with liniments written previously for contractions and spasms.

Afterward I enveloped the patient in a warm cloth, placing him on the said manure, having first garnished and covered it with white straw. Then he was very well covered with the manure. There he remained three days and nights without getting up. During this time there occurred to him a small flux of the stomach and a great sweat. Meanwhile, he began a little to open his mouth in which little by little I aided him with such an instrument which I put between his teeth.

Dilator for opening the mouth, which turns with a screw.

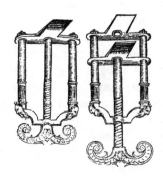

Another stronger dilator.

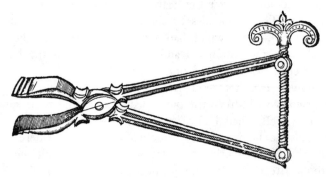

After having opened his mouth by this instrument, I put
in it a small stick of heart-pine in order that his mouth should
remain open after withdrawal of the instrument. While he
could not chew, I had him given cow's milk and soft eggs. By
this means, he was cured of the spasm. Subsequently, I followed
the cure of the arm by repeating the application of actual
cauteries on the extremity of the adjutory bone, in order always
to consume and dry the alien humidities, I must note for you
that the patient had great delight when the said cauteries were
applied to him because he said he felt a pruritus the whole
length of the adjutory bone, which was from the heat communicated by means of the cauteries, along the bone. This I
have often times seen happen at the Hostel Dieu in Paris in
similar cases. Thus great flakes or scales fell from the extremity of the bone as much from the exterior air as from the
application of the cauteries. Likewise, I fomented the part often
in order continually to dry and strengthen it, which fomentations

were made with a sour, thick, and astringent wine in which I boiled red roses, absinthe, sage, laurel, camomile flowers, and melilot, dill, and other aforesaid medicaments. By this the poor soldier was cured. Therefore, it is necessary that the surgeon have always before his eyes that God and nature command him not to leave patients without doing his duty, although he may foresee the signs of death, for nature often does what seems to the surgeon to be impossible. As very wisely one of our ancient doctors shows, saying,

Contigunt in morbis monstra, sicut et in natura.

Collection of some notable stories observed by the author. Chapter 21.

I pray the surgeons beginning to operate in the art that they do not have the wish to leave the poor languishing without treating them, this in spite of the great wounds or other dispositions contrary to nature that they may have. For often one sees many wounds and other maladies to cure after having been given up and deplored. For example, it will not grieve you if for the affection I bear you I relate to you certain other stories.

And first, when I was at Turin I was called to Montcallier to dress the wounds of a soldier named L'Evesque, native of Paris, who being then under Captain Regnoard was wounded by three great sword cuts, one of which he had in his right side over his breast, where the wound was four fingers long or about, penetrating into the capacity of the thorax. This the surgeon who first treated him had not recognized. For he would not have so indiscreetly (as I believe) sewn the wound as he did, so that nothing came out of it. This in spite of the fact that on the diaphragm had flowed a great quantity of blood which hindered the action of the diaphragm and of the lungs and consequently of the whole thorax, so that with great difficulty was he able to breathe and less to speak, having a vehement fever, his pulse very excited, and with a cough he threw out blood by the mouth, complaining of having extreme pain in his right side. The next day, as I have related, I was sent for to visit the patient and having arrived I doubted seeing such signs if he were pleuritic. As a result, I questioned the one who had treated him to know if the wound penetrated within the capacity of the thorax. He answered no. Still I dared to unsew the wound, at the orifice of which I found large clots of coagulated blood. Then quickly I had the patient raised by the legs, head down, closing his mouth and nose, in order that by this means the lungs should tumefy themselves and expel through the wound the blood contained in the thorax, in which I put my finger rather deeply through the wound, and I drew out about three saucers of coagulated blood, black, very fetid and corrupted, because it was outside its proper vessels. This done, I placed him on the bed, putting in the wound some barley water, in which I had had boiled rose honey and rock candy. Then I had the patient turned on one side and the other, in order to clean well. After this, I again had him lifted by the legs as before, then we saw come out with the blood a quantity of small clots of coagulated blood. This done, he was put on the bed where straightway the complications ceased. The following day I made injections of the aforesaid water in which I had boiled centaury, absinthe, and aloe in order better to cleanse and strengthen the part, but the patient soon after felt a marvelous bitterness in his mouth with nausea.

Then there came to my memory that I had seen at the Hostel Dieu of Paris a similar thing happen to a certain sick man who had a fistula in his thorax who demonstrated that such bitter things could be imbibed in the lungs by their thinness and sponginess, from which they were easily communicated to the windpipe and the esophagus or meri, and consequently to the mouth. Wherefore I was constrained to remove them and continue the treatment according to the doctors of our art, by which the said patient was cured.

Further, I remember having treated a servant of my lord of Champagne from the country of Anjou who was wounded by a sword cut in the throat, so that he had one of his jugular veins cut along with the windpipe. As a result, he had a very great flow of blood, besides the fact that he could not speak until his wound was sewn and dressed. And while the medicaments put on the wound were liquid, he drew them in between the stitches and gave them up through his mouth. Considering the magnitude of the wound and the nature of the parts affected, principally of the windpipe and great branches of the jugulars, which are spermatic, cold, and dry, they are for this reason difficult to reunite according to the first intention of nature. With this also is the fact that the windpipe is subject to the movement which is made in swallowing by reason of its internal tunic which is continuous with that of the esophagus, and they obey each other by a reciprocal movement as a double-headed cord in a pulley (as I have described in my *Universal Anatomy*). Considering also the use of the parts, that is, that the windpipe serves marvelously for respiration, which is necessary to the symmetry and conservation of the vital warmth to the heart, and that the jugular vein is very much required for the nutrition of the upper parts and, moreover, considering the very great quantity of blood that he had lost and was losing by the wound (which is the treasure of nature preserving the natural warmth and vital spirits) and other complications, I made a prognosis of approaching death. Still he escaped. This I believe to have rather come about by the grace of God than by the aid and means of man.

Similarly, I would give an account of many others, among whom some had had thrusts through the body and yet have recovered their health. And for the testimony of this, I have treated, in the town of Melun, the silversmith of the ambassador of the King of Portugal, who had a sword-thrust through his body by which his intestines were wounded so that when one dressed it a rather great quantity of fecal matter came out through the wound; nevertheless, the said silversmith has been cured.

And to return to our subject, I have indeed wished to recite such desperate cures to the end of always stimulating and giving courage to the surgeons who are beginning to exercise the art not to leave the grievously wounded, although they may have mortal signs, but to strive to do what the art commands, praying them not to apply themselves indifferently nor also to leave them for lack of payment, if they are indigent, but rather to aid them by a charity which we are all held by the commandment of God to exercise the one toward the other. And where one should have made some cure worthy of praise, he is not to attribute it to himself but to GOD, considering and recognizing that all good things proceed from Him, as from a fountain which cannot be exhausted, and nothing from us, as of us. Thus it is necessary to render Him thanks for all our good works, whom I entreat by all the power which is put in me by His infinite bounty, that it please Him to make us understand the cause and the end for which His divinity has given us being, to the end of not being deprived of it.

End of the book of gangrenes and mortifications.

Preface

of Book 8. on Hot-pisses.

Although my first intention was only to review my book on the wounds made by arquebuses and other firearms, in order to add to it many experiences (confirmed by very solid reasons) of the things which occurred in these last wars as much for the malignity and indisposition of the weather as for other causes amply treated in my discourse addressed to the King, and made by the command of his Majesty, which I have put at the front of this work, nevertheless, I wish for the use of the public and the instruction of young surgeons (for it is for those that I am writing) to bring to light some other little works (little, I can indeed say, for they will serve only as earnests of my general practice which I have dedicated to the King and promised to the French republic), although they have nothing in common with my first intention. I believe, however, that the addition that I have put to my first labor will not bring little fruit to our nation, considering that in the books that I have added to it I treat only of some parts of surgery, even though of the most difficult and, among others, of the cure of hot-pisses, a malady just as much troublesome to cure as it is common. This you will take as much in good part, as with good affection I desire that in the reading of my books you may profit and bear me good will for them.

The Eighth Book

speaks of the hot-pisses and strictures produced in the urinary meatus and contains 14 chapters.

TABLE OF THE CHAPTERS OF THE EIGHTH BOOK.

On the Hot Pisses

and strictures produced in the urinary meatus. Book VIII.

In what manner gonorrhea differs from hot-piss.
Chapter 1.

Some have until now thought that the hot-piss might have something in common with the gonorrhea of the ancients*, but

---

*Galen, *De Pocis Affectis*

they are very different from each other, as you will be amply able to see by this treatise. For gonorrhea is an involuntary discharge of semen, flowing from all parts of our body to the genital parts. This is done when some portion of mild and benign blood, and of the purest there is in the sanguinary mass, pellucid in color, of viscid substance, smooth and without any bad odor, falls through the passages with a small delectation, principally formed at the extremity of the staff, which anoints the passage of this against the erosion and acrimony of the urine.

On the contrary, hot-piss, or burning of urine, is a discharge which issues through the staff, of yellowish color, sometimes greenish, other times bloody, approaching the quality of a pus not well digested and of bad odor, with a sharpness which most often gnaws and ulcerates the urinary tract, making erection of the staff and of the genital parts painful. Because in the erection there is a contraction as by a particular spasm, the patients say they feel as a cord which pulls their staff downward, and such a thing is done by means of a flatulent spirit which fills the canal or cavernous nerve and the whole virile member. Because of this plethora, there is a distention of the staff which, extended in width, shows itself a little shorter.

Besides these complications, when the urinary passage is ulcerated, the patient urinating feels a grievous pain because the urine passing through the ulcers bites and stings them. Now, the flow of the discharge continues sometimes two or three years or more, which makes us believe that the hot-piss has nothing in common with gonorrhea, as we show hereafter, describing the parts which are principally affected. In addition, it is impossible that the semen could issue from the body for so long a time without its being the cause of the body's becoming languid, weak, and enfeebled (seeing that the semen is made of heavy sap from the solid parts), whence death would follow. This is indeed easy to recognize in those who have had the company of a woman five or six times, indeed less, whose body is found to be very weak and discomfited, and in some almost benumbed. Wherefore, it must be concluded that the discharge that one casts out in hot-pisses does not proceed from the sap good and dedicated to the generation of the human semen, but rather that it is a virulent, acrid, viscid, altered, and corrupted humor.

On the causes of hot-piss and differences of the same.
Chapter 2.

Hot-piss comes from three causes, that is, from too great a plethora, from too great inanition, and from contagion. That which is made by plethora is caused by a too great abundance of blood or for having been on horseback having the sun on the back, or for having used warm and flatulent foods which cause tension and heat, whence ensues inflammation of the genital parts. This makes not only the semen but also the humors flow on the said parts, principally on the prostate glands situated at the beginning of the neck of the bladder, where finish and end the spermatic vessels, of which you will find the figure and description at the end of this treatise, in order to clarify further what we tell you. Now, these prostates thereafter are abscessed and their discharge, which flows with a certain corrosion down the length of the canal of the staff, makes several ulcers in it by means of which the acrid urine passing over them bites and corrodes them further, a thing which causes a great pain in the patients, which even continues some time after having urinated. Also, in the erection of the staff, there is made a contraction (as has been said above) which proceeds from the inflammation and from the flatulent spirit which fills the cavernous nerve, by which plethora the staff swells and shortens.

That which is made by inanition comes from having too much and unreasonably used the amorous embrace, for such excess causes inflammation and by means of this an attraction of blood and of semen to the parts, which are altered and corrupted by the foreign warmth. This causes the semen to issue half formed, indeed sometimes pure blood, whence death ensues in some. Sometimes also the blood and semen are retained in the spermatic vessels because of the debilitation of the expulsive faculty, which has not the power of putting them outside, and being there, outside their proper vessels, are rotted, corrupt and wound the prostates, whence comes the hot-piss.

That which comes from contagion is made by having had the company of those who are infected by it, whether man or woman, for having cohabited with her who a little before would have received the semen of a man contaminated by the malady, who would have his purgations white, some ulcer in

157

the shameful parts, some matter proceeding from the pox, or some venomous and virulent spirit, which, insinuating itself in the genital parts, infects them and sometimes the whole body. For (as Galen shows in the third book *De Loc. Affectis*), who, seeking the truth, would believe that by the sting of a scorpion the whole body can be so strongly wounded, considering the small quantity of venom that it introduces into the body, but which nevertheless has such great power that it causes the one who is stung by it to die? Further, does not one see that by a small sting of a bee, of a wasp, or of a hornet come to pass pains, tumors, and very great inflammations? And although such stings are only superficial, their venom nevertheless can communicate its malice to the noble parts. In similar cases, it can be that the vapor of the virus of the semen or of other corrupted humors is communicated to the genital parts, principally to the prostates, which receive not only the semen, but the other humors which, putrefying, cause abscesses and ulcers from which issues a fetid and virulent pus which men throw out by the staff, and women by the neck of the womb. Sometimes also a part of the discharge falls on the testicles and on the perineum, even on the staff, which most often causes in these parts gangrenes and hollow and fistulous ulcers. Moreover, there can rise from that virus corrupted and poisonous vapors which are carried to the noble parts by the veins, arteries, and nerves, from which the pox very often proceeds.

On the prognosis of the hot-pisses. ### Chapter 3.

The hot-piss is not to be neglected, because many pernicious complications develop from it, as we have said, and it is incurable in some who cast out constantly a virulent discharge, which sometimes causes a complete suppression of urine because the prostates and the whole neck of the bladder swell and are inflamed as much by coitus as by the use of warm and vaporous foods, or by too great exercise, as is that of riding post, and also by the changing of the moons, from which suppression death ensues sometimes. Recently, I saw this happen to a certain person who, having carried a hot-piss ten years and more, kept it until death. This man, after having done some excesses, was straightway seized with a suppression of urine, by means of which he was not able to urinate without the benefit of a sound which he always carried with him. Now, not being able one day to put it as far as into the bladder, he sent for me to make him piss, which I was not able to do although I employed all the remedies possible for me, which was the cause of his death. This having occurred, I prayed his wife to permit me to open him, which she willingly granted me. I found his bladder quite full of urine and greatly distended, the prostates large, swollen, ulcerated, and quite full of pus similar to that which he cast out during his malady. Therefore, I dared to conclude that this pus which comes from the hot-pisses is made within the substance of the prostate glands and not of the kidneys (which some have thought and wished to affirm). I do not wish, nevertheless, to deny here that the kidneys may be abscessed and consumed entirely, casting out similarly a great quantity of pus. Still, the complications are not parallel to those of the hot-pisses.

Now, the ulcer which is in the neck of the bladder is easy to distinguish from that which is in the body of it because, if it is in the bladder, the discharge will be mixed with the urine and there will be in it small membranes or filaments. Its odor will be fetid and acrid, and the patient will not have as great pain. And note that I say as great because, when there is ulcer in the prostates or urinary passage, pain is always felt in the extremity of the staff, because in all extremities feeling is always more acute and exquisite, and principally so in the staff.

Now, having amply discoursed on the signs and differences of gonorrhea as well as of hot-piss, it now behooves to treat of the remedies concerning the cure of both maladies and to begin with gonorrhea.

Summary of the treatment of gonorrhea.
Chapter 4.

It is necessary to call a learned physician who will purge and bleed the patient if there is need of it and who will order him his regimen, forbidding him all things which form great quantity of blood, increase the semen, and provoke to coitus, likewise the use of wine, if it is not mean and sour, warning him to flee the frequentation of women, even of seeing them in painting or otherwise represented, particularly those for whom the patient bears some affection. Vehement exercise is good for them, and to carry heavy burdens until sweating, to bathe in cold water, to sleep little, and to apply on the loins and around the genital parts cooling and nutritive ointment of roses, then over this a large cloth soaked in oxycrate, and to renew it often, as is said hereafter. For if it is caused by debilitation of the retentive ability of the genital parts, especially for having too much used the venereal act, it is necessary to use strengthening and astringent things and above all to avoid women, indeed putting them completely in oblivion, until the patients are restored and entirely cured.

These general remedies will suffice you for the treatment of gonorrhea, seeing that the cure of this is amply treated in the learned commentaries of the physicians and surgeons, ancients as well as moderns, and also my principal intention is to give you only the remedies of hot-piss. The cure of this, in general as well as particular, will be treated below.

General treatment of hot-piss.
Chapter 5.

The cure will be changed according to the diversity of the causes and complications, for in general it is necessary for the patient to hold to a good manner of living and for him to avoid all things which heat the blood, principally all flatulent foods and violent exercises. Let him be purged and bled according to the advice of the learned physicians, principally if the ill proceeds from plethora. He is to flee the cohabitation of women (if the said hot-piss had not come from default of coitus). He is not to sleep on a feather bed but on a mattress or a soft pallet, on which one will put a cloth folded several times at the place of the region of the kidneys, and if it is possible for him he is not at all to sleep or lie on his back. He will eat his meats rather boiled than roasted, cooked with sorrel, lettuces, purslane, and some quantity of hulled barley, and of the four cold seeds crushed. For sauce, he is to content himself with juice of lemon, oranges, pomegranates, or verjuice. He will abstain from wine, in place of which he will use barley water, ptisan, broth, divine potion, or else water hippocras, with a very little cinnamon. In the morning he will take two hours before eating a hulled barley, with which he will have cooked a small linen bag full of the four cold seeds crushed, a little white poppy seed, because it refreshes, soothes, and cleanses. Likewise, he will sometimes use syrup of marshmallows or of Venus's-hair, and at times, a half-ounce of cassia alone, to which also from time to time one can add a dram of rhubarb or a half-dram in powder, according to the exigency of the case. Similarly, turpentine of Venice alone or with rhubarb in powder, or with oil of sweet almonds recently drawn and without fire, or with some of the said syrup of Venus's-hair, is a sovereign and singular remedy because it has a very great virtue of soothing and cleansing and because it aids greatly the expulsive ability to push out the virulent and infected matter contained in the prostates, considering also that because of its bitterness, it is antagonistic to putrefaction. Besides these virtues, it is of value also, due to an occult property, on the kidneys and the other parts concerned with the urine. This is recognized by its effect, as well as by the odor which it leaves in the urine after one has used it. And if there were some patients, as are found, who cannot at all take the said turpentine in bolus (in the fashion that one gives it ordinarily), it is easy to render it potable by soaking it in a mortar with a little yellow of egg and white wine, which I have learned from an apothecary who concealed this means of rendering it potable as a great secret. This I have not wished to forget to write because I know that few persons think that it can be made easy to drink, considering its viscosity and thickness. I am able to assure you that one has seen by the above remedies a great number of those sick with hot-piss recover. Nevertheless, in order to forget nothing of what we have resolved on treating, having done the general things, we shall come to the particular.

Specific treatment of hot-piss.
Chapter 6.

First, we must begin to sedate the pain and to diminish the inflammation as much as we can by making an injection into the staff of the decoction which follows:

℞ of seed of psyllium, of lettuce, of white poppy, of plantain, of quinces, of flax, of white henbane, of each ℥ ii. Let the mucores be drawn off in water of nightshade, of plantain, and of roses, as much as suffices, of Rhazes's white troches, camphorated, pulverized, ℥ i. Mix together, let it be used for injection.

This prescription written above will serve you for a formulary which you will be able to alter, increasing or diminishing it according to necessity and always guiding yourself with reason.

This injection has the power of appeasing pain because it is a refrigerant and by its viscosity lubricates and soothes the urinary canal, protecting it from the irritating and burning of the humors and from the virulent matters. One is to use the injection tepid. In place of this, one can also use milk as it comes from the cow, or else warmed a little, and especially whey or thin milk. Milk is very proper for making injection or for drinking with hot pisses and urinary burning because of the virtue that it has of refreshing and cleansing and also because it passes easily, being very subtle and thin. Externally, it will be very good to make an unction of Galen's cooling cerate, with camphor added, or of cerate of sandal, or of comitiss, or of a nutritive ointment on the region of the kidneys, on the loins, and on the perineum, even to rub with it the scrotum and the whole staff. But before using these ointments or similar ones, they must be made to melt on the fire and care taken not to cause them to heat a great deal in order that they may not lose their faculty of refrigerating, which is our principal intention.

The ointment made, it is well to apply thereon some cloths steeped in oxycrate composed of waters of plantain, of nightshade, of houseleek, or roses, and the like. In this, if it came about that the patient should have a great pain in urinating and after having urinated (which is almost ordinary), it will be good for the patient to piss in a vessel full of warm milk, soaking his staff in it during the time that he is passing his urine, and in default of milk it will be necessary to take warm water. By this remedy you will soothe a great part of the stinging. The pain mitigated by these means, you will begin to clean the ulcers of the staff by such an injection:

℞ of simple hydromel ℥ four, of syrup of dry roses, and of absinthe, of each ℥ ss. Let injection be made; let it be used for the use said.

And where there is need of greater cleansing, you will add to the injection a little Egýptiac, which I have done many times, whence thanks to God the outcome has been good. I have also seen to be of great help for this purpose the decoction which follows:

℞ of fragrant white wine lb. ss, of waters of plantain and of roses, of each ℥ ii, of orpiment ℈ i ss, of verdigris ℈ i, of Socotrine aloes ℈ iii. Let the things to be pulverized be pulverized, and let them boil together; let the decoction be used for injection.

It will be necessary for you to diminish and increase the strength of the ingredients as you see necessary.

The ulcers cleansed, it is well to use desiccation to lead them to cicatrix, drying the humor and strengthening the parts which have been permeated and relaxed by the long and extensive discharge. In order to remedy this, the decoction following is quite suitable:

℞ of forge water one pound, of rind of pomegranates and of pomegranate flowers, of crushed cypress nuts, of each ℥ one ss, of sumac and barberry, of each ℥ two, of rose syrup, and of absinthe, of each ℥ one; let decoction be made, let it be used for injection.

Some of this decoction must be thrown into the staff often with a syringe and continued until no more discharge issues. Then you can hope for the patient to be cured.

It remains now to speak of the complications which proceed from some hot-pisses, which are strictures formed in the urinary tract, by which many are tormented and, because of this, often develop a retention of urine.

On the strictures which are formed in the urinary passages after some hot-pisses. Chapter 7.

The virulent humor which issues from the prostate glands and passes continually through the canal of the staff erodes by its sharpness and ulcerates in some places the canal of the staff of men and in women the neck of the womb. Sometimes in these ulcers is formed a superfluous flesh, as we see happen in exterior ulcers, which sometimes prevents the semen and urine from passing easily by their ordinary way. From this, serious complications come to pass. Therefore, it is necessary to pay heed diligently to these ulcers, devoting oneself in full effort to cure them. In order to do this, it is important to know in the first place if they are recent or chronic, because they are so much the more troublesome to cure when they are older and more ancient, for then they are hard and callous, especially because most of the strictures have already formed scar.

On the signs of strictures. Chapter 8.

The strictures are recognized by the sound which cannot pass freely through the urinary passage but rather finds resistance as many times as there are strictures and, similarly, by the difficulty that the patient has in urinating. The urine in these maladies issues scant, forked, or askew. Sometimes it comes only drop by drop with considerable tenesmus, in the fashion that most often the patient wishing to urinate, is forced to go to the stool as those who have a stone in the bladder. Further, after he has pissed there remains a small portion of urine behind the strictures. So also does the semen after coitus, so that the patient in such case is forced to compress his staff in order to make the matters issue. Sometimes there has occurred in some an entire suppression of urine, which has caused them such a distention of the bladder that there followed from it a great inflammation and several abscesses in different places. As a result, the urine afterward issued from many places, that is, by the area around the seat, by the perineum, the scrotum, the pubes, and the groins, as I have seen in many, which is a completely incurable ill.

On the prognosis of strictures. Chapter 9.

When there is a beginning stricture, it will be well to cure it the soonest possible, for it would grow from day to day and would not at all be curable. By nature, the entire suppression of the urine and the complications above written show sufficiently the difficulty of the cure of the stricture. Furthermore, the remedies are difficult to apply to it. Nevertheless, governing yourself in general as well as in particular, as we teach you, you will be able to reach the end aimed at by you.

General observations for the cure of strictures. Chapter 10.

The time most proper for curing them is spring, and then winter. Yet, if the malady becomes urgent, one will not have consideration for the time. During the treatment, the patient is to keep himself from the venereal act, for by it the kidneys, the spermatic vessels, glands, prostates, and the whole staff swell, heat, and consequently attract from all superior parts. Thus they send to the wounded parts many excessive substances which prevent cure. Pursuing the cure of the strictures, it is well to keep from using too much acrid and corrosive remedies in the urinary passage, because the sensitivity of this passage, being injured by these, could be the cause of severe complications. It is necessary not to be afraid if from time to time some flow of blood comes from the strictures, for this is a thing quite suitable, a portion of the conjoined matter being evacuated, which even relieves the part and prevents the malady from growing, seeing that the blood is cause of the stricture. Therefore, the flow of blood not occurring of itself, it will be very well to provoke it by the sound.

Specific treatment of strictures. Chapter 11.

If the strictures are old and callous, they must be softened by fomentations, cataplasms, liniments, plasters, and fumigations. This fomentation will serve you as a form:

℞ of root of althea, and of white lilies, of each ℥ iiii, of root of bryony, and of fennel, of each ℥ i ss, of leaves of mallow, of violets, of pellitory and of mercurialis, of each m. ss, of seed of flax, of fenugreek, of each ℥ ss, juicy dried figs in number xii, of flowers of camomile, of melilot, of each p.i. Let the things to be crushed be crushed; those to be cut be cut, let all boil in ordinary water, and let fotus be made with soft female sponges. From the dregs of the said fomentation you can make a cataplasm as follows:

℞ the aforesaid materials, let them be strained, let them be pounded and spread to dry, add of hog fat cleaned of bits of skin and of basilicon ointment, of each ℥ ii; let cataplasm be made.

You will use this cataplasm after the fomentation. Between the said fomentation and application of the cataplasm you will be able to use the following liniment, or other to similar purpose:

℞ of ointment of dialthea of the description of Agrippa, of each ℥ i ss, of wool fat, and of human axunge, of each ℥ i, of fresh butter, of oil of lilies, and of camomile, of each ℥ vi. Let them be liquefied together, adding of brandy ℥ i; let liniment be made, with which you will rub the outside of the place where you think the strictures to be.

You will also be able to apply plasters tending to this same goal, and these you will prescribe as you see indicated. But if you wish to content yourself with Vigo's plaster with mercury, you will be able to do so, for I assure you that it is honored over all others for softening and destroying such hardnesses, provided that it be faithfully dispensed.

For this same purpose, you will be able to use the sub-fumigation and evaporation which follows. You must take a piece of a mill wheel (for we use this stone in the place of that which the ancients have named pyrites) or you will take large bricks and, having heated them well in the fire, you will put them in a copper basin or a small cauldron beneath a closed stool. Then the patient, being seated on the stool as if he wished to go to his affairs, you will pour on the said stones some good vinegar and some brandy mixed together in equal parts, and you will garnish the said chair so well around that the vapor is not lost, rather that it is carried straight against the malady.

In order to do still better, you will be able to use this cask, within which the patient will be nude and seated in the middle on a board with a hole at the place of the genital parts. Then there will be a cauldron between his legs in which one will put the heated stones, and through the little window marked B, you will sprinkle the said stones with the abovesaid liquid, the fumes of which the patient will receive conveniently on the affected part. It is necessary that the patient be well enclosed and covered in the cask marked A and that the little window be similarly well closed, for fear that the vapor may be lost.

Cask proper for receiving a fumigation.

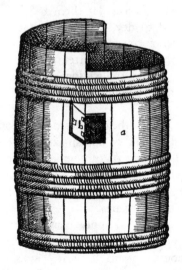

166

Such evaporation penetrates, cuts, dissolves, liquefies, softens, and dissolves greatly all scirrhous hardnesses, witness Galen.

Those remedies that must be used if the said strictures result from pox. Chapter 12.

But if there is suspicion that the hardness and strictures are caused by some humor resulting from pox, the patient must diet and use a decoction of guaiac, rubbing his groin, all the perineum, and the staff with an ointment proper to pox. For otherwise, one would lose the trouble and his time. While he is in a sweat, it will be well to have him hold between his legs a bottle filled with boiling water, or a hot brick, well enveloped in cloths sprinkled in vinegar and brandy, because by means of these stones there will rise a vapor and warmth which, along with ointment for the pox, will soften and melt the humor causing the strictures. This I have practiced in many with very good outcome.

How it is necessary to proceed in curing the softened strictures. Chapter 13.

After having by these means thus softened the strictures, it is necessary to consume them with remedies which have the power of destroying them. And if one recognizes that they are callous and have taken cicatrix (which will be easy to see because no excessive moisture will issue from them), then it becomes necessary to excoriate them and break them with a sound or rod of lead having, one finger's breadth from its extremity, many unevennesses as does a round file. Having passed it in the staff beyond the strictures, the patient or the surgeon will pull it, push it back, and turn it as many times as he will see in his opinion to be necessary in order to destroy and comminute the strictures, letting flow afterward a rather good quantity of blood in order always to purge the part. One will also be able to use several sounds proper for such purpose, within which there will be a silver wire, and at the extremity of this a small roundness which will be sharp and hollow toward the end of the sound. This is so that it may join closely in order to put it into the staff without violence, at the place of the strictures, and then one will push the staff against the sound as much or as little as one will wish. And having thus pushed it, one withdraws it as many times as one wishes. Doing this, one pinches and comminutes from the stricture as much as seems to be good for one time. I can assure you that I have made fine cures by it. The cannula marked a. is similarly useful for such effect. Its use is such: It is necessary to put it in the staff, and its openings marked b.b. serve for cutting and comminuting the strictures when they are placed inside, and then one is to turn the cannula and compress with the fingers at the place on the staff where the strictures are.

Sounds and cannula proper for cutting and comminuting strictures.

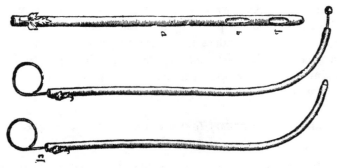

Afterward it will be necessary to use the following powder, which, because of the ingredients, holds the first place among all the remedies proper for consuming the strictures and excresences of flesh in the shameful parts, in man as well as in woman, without notable pain:

℞ of savin dried in the shade ℥ ii, of ochre, of antimony, of prepared tutty, of each ℥ ss. Let fine powder be made, as alcohol.

It is necessary to apply this powder with the abovesaid cannula and with a small silver rod, which will be in proportion to the cavity of the cannula, at the end of which you will have bound a small piece of soft cloth, and the cannula being put with the window upward, in order that the powder will not fall into the urinary passage. You will direct the window on the stricture, for by pushing with the rod, you will push the powder out of the cannula. Then afterward you will withdraw the cannula, having turned the window around on the other side from the stricture, in order not to carry powder back into the window but rather so that it remain on the stricture the longest time that it will be possible. And if great pain occurs, it is well to use the following injection to mitigate the pain and to force out inflammation:

℞ of juices of purslane, of plantain, of nightshade, and of houseleek, of each ℥ ss, whites of eggs in number vi, let them be stirred a long time in a leaden mortar, and tepid let them be injected into the staff through the fistula.

You can in place of this one use the injection that we have written heretofore in the chapter of the special cure of hot-piss. There will be need also to put outside the length of the genital parts some repellent remedies to prevent pain and inflammation. One can likewise use remedies which have the faculty of diminishing and dissolving strictures, among which the following are very excellent:

℞ of prepared tutty ℨ vi, of antimony ℨ iii, of Rhazes's white troches camphorated ℨ i, of rind of pomegranates, of burnt alum, of each ℨ i ss, of burnt sponge ℈ ii. Let all be pulverized very finely, as alcohol. Afterward:

℞ of diapompholigos ointment and of Rhazes's white ointment, of each ℥ ii. Let them be mixed with the aforesaid powders in a leaden mortar, and let them be stirred for a long time.

This ointment will be applied with a small candle of wax or a sound wrapped in a very delicate cloth, which will remain in the staff by turning the sound or candle in the other direction from that in which it will have been wrapped and covered. Then you will withdraw the said cloth by an end which will pass the staff and you will see at the place where the cloth covered with ointment touched the strictures the operation of the remedy. One can also use other candles of wax, the wick of which will be made expressly of very strong and delicate thread for fear that they may break, but it is necessary that at the place where they will touch the strictures, they be formed and extended by the composition which follows:

℞ of black plaster or of diachylon with iris ℥ ii, of powder of beans, of ochre, of calcined Roman vitriol, of powder mercurialis, of each ℨ ss. Let all be liquefied together for the use said.

This remedy can be increased in its force or diminished as the surgeon recognizes to be necessary. When one uses the above remedies, it is necessary to take care that the patient shake his staff well and that he endeavor that not a drop of urine remain in the urinary passage after he has pissed, for it is not possible for so little of it to remain that it would not prevent the action of the above remedies.

On the remedies suitable to cicatrize the ulcers after the ablation of the strictures. Chapter 14.

After the stricture is destroyed by these remedies, which one can recognize when the patient pisses freely and at ease and as heavily as he had been accustomed before he was sick, and, likewise, when on putting the sound into the passage one does not feel any hindrance, it is then necessary to dry and cicatrize the ulcer, which one will be able to do with such and similar injection, which has great virtue of drying and cicatrizing without much biting, as one will recognize by its ingredients:

℞ of forge water lb. ss, of cypress nuts, of galls, of rind of pomegranates, of each ℈ i ss, of rock alum ℈ ss. Let all boil together according to the art; let decoction be made for the injection.

This, one will use until one perceives no discharge to issue from the staff. Similarly, in order to dry further and to advance the cicatrization, it will be good to use this powder, which dries without any pain and biting:

Take washed calaminary stone, burnt egg shells, red coral, rind of pomegranate, and the whole powdered finely. Then let them be applied on the ulcers with candles of wax, anointed with ointment of red desiccative, or other similar. For the same effect, one will use rods or sounds of lead, the thickest that the patient can endure, and put these in the staff as far as the ulcers, having first rubbed them with quicksilver, and hold them there night and day as long a time as the patient will be able. They have the virtue of drying, cicatrizing, and dilating the urinary passage without any pain. I could further write you a large booklet of remedies tending to similar goal as those written above but, knowing well that the expert surgeon can change and vary them by reason, as the malady requires, these will serve you as examples.

And because I had heretofore promised you to give you the description and figure of the bladder, prostates, and other parts necessary for the intelligent use of this treatise, I have, to acquit myself of my promise, drawn from my *Universal Anatomy* these two figures, the parts of which are described to you by letters as follows:

Description of the figure of the anterior part.

A   Demonstrates the hollow vein [vena cava].

B   The great artery [aorta].

CC The emulgent veins and arteries, entering into the kidneys.

DD The ureters.

EE The spermatic veins.

FF The spermatic arteries.

G   The place where the great artery rides on the great vein [vena cava], in order not to be compressed by the sacrum.

H   The junction and mingling of the seminal vein and artery, degenerating into varicose texture, ending in the membrane named epididymis.

II   The two testicles.

KK Expellant or ejaculatory vessels [vas deferens].

L   The anterior part of the body of the bladder.

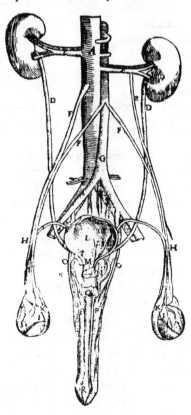

Figure of the anterior part.

171

M   The orifice and beginning of the neck of the bladder.

NN The anterior face of the two prostate glands, of which we have here made so much mention and in which principally hot-piss is made.

OO Veins and arteries which descend from the beginning of the neck of the bladder to the extremity of the staff.

PP Two spongy ligaments of which the staff is composed.

Q   The canal common to the urine as well as to the sperm in which the ulcers of hot-piss are made.

R   The glands, which is the end and extremity of the staff.

Description of the posterior part.

A   Shows the great artery.

B   The hollow vein.

DD The vessels emulgent to the kidneys.

EE The ureters with their entry into the bladder.

FF The spermatic veins.

GG Spermatic arteries.

HH The varicose vessels.

II The testicles.

KK The varicose prostates making the ejaculatory vessels [vas deferens].

LL The junction and concurrence of the expellant vessels [vas deferens], passing within the prostates to go to the channel of the neck of the bladder.

MM The two glands named heretofore prostates.

N   The muscle named sphincter which is in the neck of the bladder, of which we shall speak amply hereafter when we treat the manner of drawing out the stone.

OO The spongy ligaments separated from their origin, which is in the inferior part of the pubis.

P   The common canal of the urine and of the semen in which strictures are formed.

Friend reader, you are not to find it strange if I have entirely exposed these two figures to you, although some of the parts of these do not appertain to this matter. Nevertheless, in order to show you that I have at all times devoted myself to the service of the public good, and also in order that you might have clearer intelligence of that of which I have spoken above, I have given you an entire description of it, because doing otherwise and giving you to understand by the letters only that which served for the matter treated heretofore, you would have had defective and half-useless figures. Besides this, the knowledge of the connection of the parts does a great deal for treating the complications of the maladies which occur in these. Thus, may it suffice you of the cure of hot-pisses and strictures.

End of Book 8 on the hot-pisses.

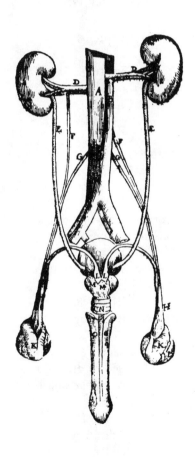

Figure of the posterior part.

The Ninth Book

is on the stones which are engendered in the bladder and in the kidneys and contains 18 chapters.

TABLE OF THE CHAPTERS OF THE NINTH BOOK

On the Stones

which are formed in the bladder and in the kidneys. Book IX.

On the cure of the stones.
Chapter 1.

The stones which are made in the bladder most often take their origin from the kidneys and descend into the bladder by the urinary vessels. The cause of this is double, that is, material and efficient. The material causes are heavy, sticky humors, thick and viscid, formed from crudities caused by poorly regulated temperature and immoderate exercises, principally suddenly after the meal, and for this cause children are more subject to this malady than the older, as one sees by experience.

The efficient cause is excessive warmth, which consumes the thin serosity, and that which is more earthy remains and dries, as we see done in tiles and bricks, of which the fire consuming the moisture, the rest turns into stone. What aids a great deal in this are the too-narrow urinary passages and

175

channels, so that the thick and viscid excrements can not pass and be cast out by these but rather remain in the substance of the kidneys or of the bladder. Then they are amassed, the ones on the others. Thus by accretion is made a stone as by scale. And just as the candler dipping his wick several times in tallow makes of it a thick candle, likewise the most crass and viscid part of the urine in passing over a little gravel or stone adheres to it and encrusts itself; then through some space of time it grows larger and makes a large stone.

On the signs of stones in the kidneys.
Chapter 2.

The signs of the stones formed in the kidneys* are that the patient casts out with the urine red or yellowish sands and he feels dull pruritus in the kidneys with gravity and heaviness of the loins. When he moves, he suffers a sharp pain and numbness or formication in the loins, hips, and thigh, because the stone, being enclosed in the kidney or in the ureteral orifice, presses the nerves proceeding from the vertebrae of the loins.

On the signs of stones in the bladder.
Chapter 3.

One will recognize the stone in the bladder by these signs, that is, that the patient feels a heaviness (that is, if it is large) in the seat and perineum, with jactitative and sharp pain, which extends to the extremity of the staff, so that he keeps on pulling and rubbing it, whence it becomes elongated and relaxed beyond measure, and most often stiff. For with the pain that he suffers is a great desire to piss, but he can not quite freely and sometimes pisses only drop by drop. And in urinating he feels an extreme pain, crossing his legs and sitting on the ground with cries and groaning and very great tenesmi, because the stone is a thing foreign to nature. Therefore, the explusive virtue strives to cast it out, which causes the tenesmi, and by these often the muscle of the seat name sphincter is relaxed. Then a portion of the straight intestine issues outside, and similarly tenesmi come to some, and hemorrhoids with extreme pain.

In addition, in the bottom of their urine is found a thick, viscid, and adhering humor, sometimes as thick as small oysters

*Hippocrates, *Epidemiques*

or as white of egg. Such a thing shows that the stone is made by diminution of natural warmth. Further, the patient has a pale, yellowish, or livid color, his eyes are dull, and he is not able to sleep or drink except with great difficulty because he is in almost continual pain.

Moreover, one will know by the sound. Have the patient stand, a little bent forward, his legs distant the one from the other by a foot or about, and let him be supported from behind. Then one will apply one of these sounds (such as there will be need), first anointed with oil or butter, passing it dexterously as far as inside the capacity of the bladder, if it is possible. And where by such position, one cannot put the sound in the bladder, it will behoove to place the patient on the edge of his bed, leaning backward a little, his knees bent, and his heels near his buttocks, as you can see in the figure depicted hereafter of those from whom one draws the stone by incision. Doing this, one will more easily put the sound within the bladder, and by it one will feel the stone by a resistance and hardness of a hard body with a dull sound at the end of the sound, which will cause one to judge correctly that there is truly a stone in it.

And you will note here for a precept, that among all the above signs, that of the sound is the most certain for knowing if there is a stone or not. The sounds will be curved, and the surgeon will have some of different lengths and thicknesses, for the diversity of the bodies. Further, when one puts them into the bladder to make them urinate, it is necessary to put in a small silver wire to prevent any humor or blood from choking it at the end, which would be cause that the urine could not pass through, and when it is in the bladder, one is to withdraw the silver wire in order that the urine may pass freely through it.

The figure of the sounds and of the silver wire is such:

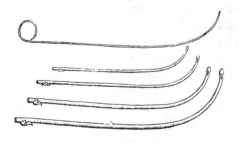

177

On the prognosis of stones.
Chapter 4.

The stone, having issued from one of the kidneys and stopped in its ureter, stops it up completely, nevertheless, the patient will not leave off urinating because, nature having made our body double, the urine will regurgitate and will be voided by the other ureter. And if such a complication happens to both, the urine will be completely suppressed, which will be the cause of the death of the patient. In dying, he will make similar aspirations as those who are drowning in a great water, for the reason that the urine overflows within the great hollow vein and consequently in the others, and they die, because the natural warmth is suffocated and extinguished by the too great quantity of urine. Those in whom nature casts some small stone of the kidneys and it stops in the ureteral vessels, some causing an extreme pain until they have descended into the bladder, have several complications, as tenesmi and desire of going to the stool and of urinating, and do not because they are most often constipated by flatulence, the proof of which is that they belch almost continually. And if the patient sneezes or coughs, or if he makes any great commotion of the body, he feels a sharp pain (principally if the stone is horned and if it has rough edges) in the place where the stone is arrested. Similarly, the pain is communicated to the hip and the thigh, and to some it seems to them that one is pulling their testicles upward with great violence. Further, they are vexed by colic with bilious vomitings and generalized sweats.

The stone is more often formed in the kidneys of the old than it is in the young for the reason that their expulsive faculty is weaker. On the contrary, it is formed in the bladder of the young more often than in the old, inasmuch as their natural warmth is stronger and, consequently, their expulsive faculty is more vigorous, and also because they are more immoderate, as we have said heretofore. When it is in the bladder and the patient casts out blood with the urine, it is a sign that the stone is neither large nor smooth but, on the contrary, is small and horned, or spiny, that is to say, with rough surfaces. For the smaller it is, the more easily it enters into the neck and orifice of the bladder, and by this means there is more difficulty in its being driven back from it and re-entering without doing violence because it scratches and ulcerates the parts where such rough surfaces touch, which is the cause of casting out blood by the staff. Also, when the urine is white and milky, it is a sign that the stone is smooth. Likewise, the patient does not feel such pain as when it has rough surfaces. And if the stone, being in the kidneys, is spiny, he will feel pricking pain as of stings, not being able to bend or move except with difficulty if he works. He casts out a sanguinous urine, indeed sometimes quite pure blood, because of the violence that it does against the walls of the channels in which it has been formed.

Now, the stones which are formed in the kidneys will be large and small and of diverse forms and figures, by reason of the interceptions in the small ventricles which are in the depth of the cavities of the channels. Truly, I have found in some after their death stones large as the finger and of the figure of a greyhound, other times of a pig, other times round and smooth, other times square, and with many rough edges, as a pine cone, other times a single one, other times many and of different colors, as black, yellowish, whitish, reddish, ashy, and others of different forms and colors, according to the temperament of the patients. In the choleric and lean, the stones are commonly made by warmth and foreign dryness, and in the phlegmatic and fat by coldness and congelation and by obstruction of the meatuses.

Sometimes the stone falls from the bottom of the bladder to the urinary passage and completely stops it up, and then there occurs entire suppression of urine. Then it is necessary to place the patient on his back and raise his legs in the air, agitating and shaking him as if one wanted to ensack something in a bag, in order to push the stone back out of the urinary passage. And likewise, it can be pushed back with a sound.

Those who have the stone in the kidneys or in the bladder are in almost continual pain. However, to some their pain comes by paroxysms, and they will be sometimes a month or two, more or less, indeed an entire year, without feeling pain. Those who have stones in the kidneys most often make clear urines. Women are not so subject to engendering stones as men because the neck of the bladder is shorter and more wide, lax, and ample. Therefore, when there is a beginning of stone, it issues forth before it is very large. Nevertheless, in some they are formed and grow as much as in men, whence it is well to incise them and aid them by similar remedies as one does in men.

When the stone exceeds the largeness of an egg in men, most often pulling it lacerates the body of the bladder. And if such a thing is done, the urine will flow involuntarily forever, because the bladder is nervous and bloodless. Therefore, it can not consolidate itself or reunite, and further most often there occurs in it inflammation and subsequently death. Stones moderately large are drawn out more safely, and the patient escapes more quickly than if they were small, for the reason that the said patient is long accustomed to patience, tolerating ordinarily inflammation, pain, and other complications, which is not the same in the others. If the stone adheres strongly to the bladder and is covered with a membrane, wishing to draw it out, one lacerates the bladder and from this ensue convulsions, gangrene, and subsequently death. You are to note here that the stone, being thus covered by a membrane, is difficult to find with the sound. In addition, if the stone is of long shape, and one takes it crosswise, one will lacerate and will break the bladder, whence will ensue the aforesaid complication. If the surgeon by chance pinches the body of the bladder with his instruments and lacerates it and separates it from the parts where it is joined, there will ensue convulsion and other aforesaid complications. Now, because it will be separated from the parts to which it adheres, great inflammation will be made because of the blood which will flow between these parts and will putrefy, following the aphorism of Hippocrates who said, "If blood is shed in the belly unnaturally, it inevitably putrefies." Therefore will follow also gangrene, mortification, and subsequently death.

After having thus written the causes of the stones which are found in the body, the manner by which they are formed, the signs of the places where they are, the symptoms and the complications, and the prognosis, at present it is necessary to write about the treatment that is conservative and curative and how it is necessary to diversify the remedies and instruments according to the bodies and parts where they are found.

On the conservative cure.
Chapter 5.

The conservative cure will be made by ordering the regimen on the six non-natural things, avoiding the causes of the gross and viscid humors. Then, to instruct you of it summarily, it is necessary to avoid dwelling in a heavy and vaporous air. As for the diet, it is necessary to avoid fish, meat of beef, of pork, river birds, vegetables, cheeses, milk products, fried and hard eggs, rice, pastries, unleavened bread, and generally all other foods which make obstruction. Also, it is necessary to guard oneself from eating garlics, onions, leeks, mustard, spices, and generally all things which warm the blood, and principally those in whom one will have conjectured that the cause of the stone is made by excessive warmth. And as for their drink, they must abstain from bad, brackish, and muddy waters, and from thick unsettled wines, beers, and other similar beverages. Further, he must not eat too much nor gluttonously for fear that he may engender in himself crudities and consequently obstructions. Sleeping soon after the meal is very harmful because it engenders crudities. Too much staying awake, working, and fasting are also harmful because they inflame the blood and so are also cause of indigestion and of foreign warmth.

If there is congestion, it is necessary to void by medicaments and phlebotomy, as well as by vomiting, which is a singular remedy for prevention of the stone. It is necessary also not to neglect the passions of the spirit. And for the evacuation of the crass and viscid humors, you will be able to have the counsel of the learned physician. Still considering that one cannot always get a physician, I have indeed wished to describe for you here some good and approved remedies which you will be able to use as you will see there is need. Here you will note for a precept of Galen* who has commanded that it is necessary to avoid diuretic things and strong purgations when there is inflammation in the kidneys and in the bladder, because they would increase it, making the humors flow in greater abundance, which would be cause of increasing the pain and other complications. Therefore, it will be necessary to use in such cases cooling and softening things internally, as well as externally, as this syrup:

℞ of tips of mallow, of marshmallow and of violariae, of each m. ss, of root of althea ℥ i, of scraped licorice ℥ iii ss, of the four greater cold seeds, of each ℥ i. Let decoction be made; take of the aforesaid decotion lb. ss, and in the straining dis-

_____

*Method, bk. XIII

181

solve of whitest sugar lb. ss, of white honey gill i. Let syrup be made according to the art, which the patient will be able to use often. Also he will use now and then a half-ounce of freshly cleaned cassia, with one dram or a dram and a half or two drams of powdered rhubarb, according to need, one hour before his meal. You will also be able to use this other concoction with great effect:

℞ of root of asparagus, of graminis of polypody of oak, of cleaned raisins, of each ℥ ss, of betony, of herniosa, of agrimony, of ominum capill, of Alexandrine laurel, of each m. ss, of the four greater cold seeds, of seed of fennel, of each ℨ i, of leaves of senna ℨ vi. Let decoction be made to lb. ss, in the straining let be dissolved of syrup of althea and of herniosa, of each ℥ i ss; let very clear and very aromatic apozem be made with a very little cinnamon for two doses; let him take the first dose in the morning two hours before his meal, and the other at four in the afternoon.

Also, at times he will use the following broth, which is of marvelous effect. Take a capon and a knuckle of veal cooked in water with a handful of hulled barley, roots of parsley, sorrel, fennel, chicory, butcher's broom, of each a half-ounce, at the end one will add leaves of sorrel, purslane, lettuce, tips of mallow, March violets, of each a half-handful, and then the broth will be kept. Of this the patient will take for four mornings two hours before eating the quantity of a half-pint with two fingers of juice of lemon, making it boil to bubbling before each taking, and shortly one will see a marvelous operation, for by the urine one will see gravels and great quantity of crass and viscid matter. Therefore, it demonstrates by its effect that it cleans and expels the matters from the parts dedicated to the urine and does no harm to the stomach or to the other parts through which it passes. I can say that it is a medical food.

You will also be able to use the following powder with great profit:

℞ of nucleorum medlars ℨ i, of powder of electuary, of cold diatragacanth ℥ ii, of the four greater cold seeds, cleaned, of scraped licorice, of each ℨ i, of seed of saxifrage ℨ ii, of seeds of gromwell, of genista, of Alexandrine laurel, of butcher's broom and of asparagus, of each Ɵ i, of seed of althea ℨ i ss, of rock candy ℥ i ss., of whitest sugar ℥ vi. Let powder be made.

It is necessary to use this powder the first day of the new moon, of the first quarter of the full moon, and of the last quarter, and all the following months, and take of it the quantity of a spoonful in the morning three hours before eating. Further, the patient will be able to use a clyster such as this one:

℞ of lettuce, of endive, of leaves of willow, of purslane, of each m. i, of flowers of violets and of nenuphar, of each p. ss. Let decoction be made to lb. i. In the straining dissolve of cassia fistula ℥ i, of violet honey and red sugar of each ℥ i, of violet oil ℥ iii. Let a clyster be made which one will give with a syringe similar to this one rather than with the clyster bag of the ancients.

Syringe for clyster.

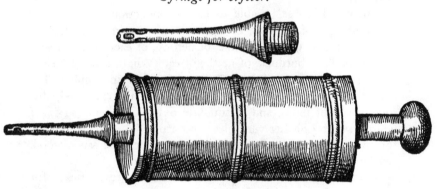

Another syringe for a woman who would be shameful, who could give herself the clyster.

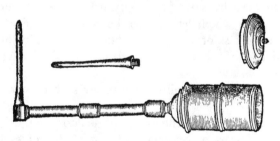

Another to calm the pain similarly:

℞ of flowers of camomile, of melilot, of tips of dill, of anagallis, of each p. ii. Let decoction be made in cow's milk, and in the straining dissolve of cassia fistula and of white sugar ℥ i,

yolks of eggs in number iii, of oil of dill and camomile, of each
℥ ii. Let clyster be made.

Outside on the kidneys and lengthwise one will apply rose
ointment nutritive, or populeon ointment alone or mixed together,
then on top a napkin steeped in oxycrate. Now if the formation
of the stone occurs by frigidity, it is necessary to relieve it by
contrary things, whence it will be necessary to use the following
remedy:

℞ of old theriac ℨ i, of rind of lemon ℨ ii, of cooked water
℥ i ss. Mix, let potion be made.

Another potion: ℞ of freshly extracted cassia ℨ vi, of herb
bennet ℨ iiii, of water of fennel ℥ ii, of water of asparagus
℥ i ss. Let potion be made; let him take it iii hours before
luncheon.

He will likewise be able to use a concoction:

℞ of root of cyperus, of burdock, of gramin, of each ℨ iii,
of marshmallow with the whole, of betony, of each m. ss, of seed
of gromwell, of burdock, of nettle, of each ℨ ii, of seed of melon,
of scraped licorice, of each ℨ ii ss, figs, iiii in number. Let
decoction be made to three gills, strained and expressed, dissolve syrup of radish and of squillitic oxymel, of each ℥ i ss, of
whitest sugar ℥ iii. Let very clear and aromatic apozem be made
for three doses with cinnamon and ℨ ss of citrine sandalwood.
Let be taken ℥ iiii three hours before luncheon.

Further, one can use this powder which has great efficacy for
dissipating the material of the calculus:

℞ of seed of parsley and of its cleaned root, of each ℨ iiii,
of seed of the thistle which is called star-thistle, ℥ i. Let them be
dried in an oven by slow fire, afterward let them be pounded
separately, with which let powder be made, of which let the
patient take ℈ i ss or ℈ ii with white wine or with broth of
young chicken, of which let the patient drink three days on an
empty stomach.

Likewise, the patient will be able to use such clysters against
flatulence:

℞ of mallow, of marshmallow, of pellitory, of origan, of
calamint, of flowers of camomile, of tips of dill, of each m. i,
of anise, of caraway, of cumin, of fennel, of each ℥ ss, of bays
of laurel ℨ iii, of seed of rue ℨ ii. Let decoction be made; in
the straining dissolve of herb bennet or of diaphenicum* ℥ ss, of

---

*Cotgrave: "a purging electuary made of the dates called Phenices"

184

confection of bays of laurel ℥ iii, of red sugar ℥ i, of oils of dill, camomile, rue, of each ℥ i. Let clyster be made.

Another easy to make for the same purpose:

℞ of oil of nuts, of malmsey wine, of each lb. ss.

If one is to hold them as long as one will be able, they will do a better operation and will appease the pains better. By the above means, one can prevent the formation of the stones and relieve also the pain of the windy colic as well as the nephritic.

On the means of succoring him who has a stone in one of the ureters, descended from the kidney. Chapter 6.

Having spoken enough of the conservative cure of the stone, it remains for us to pursue the means for relieving those who are afflicted by it in the kidneys, ureters, as well as in the bladder. In the first place, we shall speak of a patient who has a stone passed from one of the kidneys which remained in one or the other of the ureters and whose urine might be suppressed wholly or in part. Then the patient feels great pain in the place where it has remained, and by a feeling in the vicinity of the hip, bladder, testicles, and in the staff with a wish to urinate, and to go to the stool. To make it descend, it is necessary (if it is possible for the patient) that he mount on a trotter or curtal, and that he ride it a league, more or less, for by this equitation and movement the stone descends into the bladder. Where he will not have the means of riding a horse, he must go up and down a staircase several times until he is weary and in sweat, and then he must be given to drink things which anoint, soften, and relax, such as recently drawn oil of sweet almonds, with water of pellitory, and white wine. Also, one is to make frictions with warm linen cloths sliding downward and to apply cupping glasses with great flames, of which you see the portrait here:

And they are to be applied now on the loins, now on the belly, pulling toward the groin a little below the pain, in order always to attract the stone into the bladder. If the patient does not vomit, it is necessary to provoke him to do this by giving him to drink water and warm oil in sufficient quantity, for vomiting helps a great deal to drive the stone downward because of the compression of the parts in such action. And

Large, medium, and small cupping glasses.

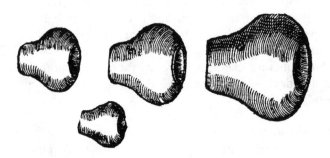

if by such remedies the patient is not relieved, it is necessary to put him in a demi-bath made of the decoction which follows:

℞ of mallow, of marshmallow with the whole, of each m. ii, of betony, of nasturtium and of anagallis, of saxifrage, of pellitory, of violariae, of each m. iii, of seed of melon, of gromwell, of alkekengi, of each ℥ vi, of red chick-peas lb. i, of root of celery, of gramin. of fennel and of eryingo, of each ℥ iiii. Let all be boiled down in sufficient quantity of water for immersion.

All of these things will be put in a sack on which the patient will be seated, and let him soak as far as the navel. And he must not remain in it as far as extreme feebleness, for by the baths is made great dissolution of the spirits and weakening of the strength. Such baths quiet the pain, relax all the parts, and open and dilate the urinary passages. In doing this, often times the stone descends into the bladder. Where the stone by such means is not displaced and there is entire suppression of urine, and also when before the bath one would not have known how to pass the sound into the bladder, it is necessary again to sound it on leaving the bath, because then the sound will enter it more easily than before. Further, it is necessary for the patient to guard himself well from the cold. You will be able by this figure to know the fashion of the demi-bath.

Description of the demi-bath chair.

a. The chair.
b. The hole in this, where the patient is seated.

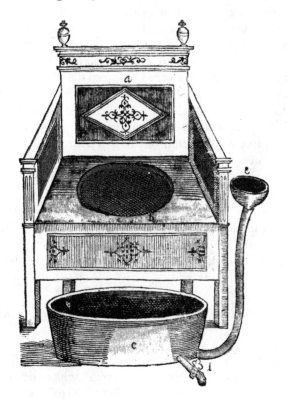

c. The tub in which the water is put.
d. The fountain for emptying the water when it is too cold.
e. The funnel by which one puts in warm water.

Another decoction for making a demi-bath:

℞ of root of radish, of althea, of each lb. ii, of root of
butcher's broom, of parsley and of asparagus, of each lb. i, of
cimini, of sweet fennel, of ammi, of each ℥ iiii, of seed of flax
and of fenugreek, of each ℥ vi, of flowers of camomile, of melilot,
of dill, of leaves of horehound, of pellitory, of each m. ii. Let
all boil together according to the art with sufficient water and a
little odoriferous white wine as far as the consumption of the
third part, and let sitz bath be made.

Further, it is useful to make with this decoction a clyster
with oil of lily ℥ iiii. and two yellows of egg. When one

wishes to give it to the patient, in the clyster bag or tube, one will add to it a half-ounce of oil of juniper, assuring yourself that it quiets promptly the pain caused by flatulence. Here it must be noted that in the great nephritic pains, it is necessary not to give too great quantity of decoction for fear that the too-filled intestines may compress the kidneys and ureteral orifices, which have already begun to be inflamed, because by that the pain would be increased and other complications would be provoked. In addition, one can apply such a cataplasm on the place of the pain, on the perineum, and on the genital parts, which has great power of calming the pain and helping to make the stone descend from the ureters into the bladder:

℞ of root of althea, of radish, of each ℥ iiii, of pellitory, of fennel, of groundsel, of nasturtium, of anagallis, of each m. i, of rupturewort m. ss, all cooked sufficiently in water, then pounded, add of oil of dill, of camomile, of rabbit grease, of each ℥ iii, flour of chick-peas as much as suffices; let cataplasm be made for the use said.

How it is necessary to proceed to the cure of the stone that has descended into the bladder. Chapter 7.

If the stone has fallen into the bladder and if there is only one (for often times there are several which descend with a multitude of gravel or sand), then the pain ceases and the patient will feel pruritus with a little stinging in the extremity of the staff. Then, if he is not weak, he must work on foot or on horseback, and he must use such a powder:

℞ of powder of lithontriptic electuary ℥ iiii, let be taken ℨ i three hours before luncheon as well as before dinner with white wine or with broth of red chick-peas.

And it is necessary that he drink good wine in rather good quantity and that he retain his urine long if he can, in order that the great mass of this drive and push the stone out of the bladder more easily. Likewise, he must be given such an injection:

℞ of syrup of Venus's-hair ℥ i, of water of alkekengi ℥ iii, of oil of scorpions ℥ ss. and some of this will be injected into his bladder with a syringe of such fashion:

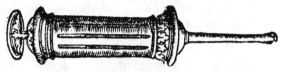

On the stone's being in the passage of the staff,
or in the neck of the bladder. Chapter 8.

If stone has come out of the body of the bladder and has remained in its neck or in the staff, then it is necessary for the surgeon to guard himself well from pushing it back in, but he will move it as much as can be done with his fingers to the extremity of the staff by injecting in it oil of sweet almonds or other lubricative things. And if it descends as far as the extremity of the staff and remains there, it must be drawn out with little hooks such as you see in this figure:

Little hooks proper for extracting a small stone
remained in the extremity of the staff.

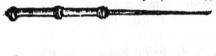

If one can not extract it by such little hooks, one will put this instrument named terebra with its cannula (approaching the figure of the extractor of arquebus balls, described heretofore, but it is not as thick or as long) into the staff as far as the stone. Then one will turn it gently in order that it may comminute the stone and make it into small portions, which will be done easily because the terebra has its extremity in the manner of a gimlet.

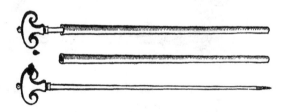

And it must be noted that it is not to be thicker than a large sound, in order that it may not do any violence in putting it into the staff.

On the means that must be used to draw out by incision a stone arrested in the urinary tract that one has not been able to extract by the above ways. Chapter 9.

Moreover, when the stone is so large or has a rough surface and is far from the extremity of the staff so that it might not be drawn out and the urine is suppressed, then it is necessary to make an incision (which I have done many times) in the side of the staff, and not on top, nor underneath; not on top, because of a large vein and artery which could be cause of flow of blood. Underneath is not suitable because the part is bloodless, and for this reason difficult to consolidate and also because the urine would not permit the union to be made because it would pass through the ulcer and would fall between the lips of the wound. For these reasons, the incision will be made on the stone in the side (which is a fleshier part). But you are to note here that, before making the incision, you must bind the staff above and quite near the stone, in order to hold it constrained and subject. Then pull the prepuce toward you rather strongly in order that after the incision, the skin, being relaxed, may return and cover the said incision, whence more easily and briefly the union and consolidation afterward will be made. Afterward you will draw the stone out by such an instrument:

Instruments proper for extracting the stone after the incision of the staff.

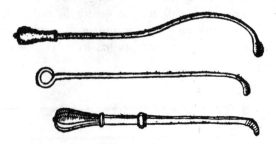

How it is necessary to treat the wound, the incision made. Chapter 10.

Then, if there is need, one will use a stitch to reunite the wound, and on it one will apply such an agglutinative:

℞ of Venice turpentine ℥ iii, of gum elemi ℥ i, of dragon's

blood and of mastic, of each 3 ss. Let medicine be made for the use said.

And around the whole staff it will be necessary to put such a repellent:

℞ of whites of eggs with powder of Armenian bole, aloes, of volatile flour, of rose oil.

Then it is necessary to continue the rest of the cure as of other wounds made in the fleshy parts. Also, one will put within the staff a candle of wax or a rod of lead anointed with Venice turpentine to aid nature to agglutinate the wound and to hold the canal smooth and equally dilated in this place, for fear that some superfluous flesh might be made, from which then afterward could be formed a stricture.

On the manner of drawing out by incision the stones which are in the bladder of a small male child. Chapter 11.

After having thus written of the means by which the small stones are extracted, now it is necessary to show by method how the large can be and are to be drawn out of the body of the bladder, and by what instruments. And we will begin with the small children, then with the men, and subsequently with the women.

Having then supposed that we have a young child to be incised, the surgeon must first make him jump five or six times in order to make the stone descend downward. Then he will place him on the knees of a man seated on a stool, on whose knees there will be a cloth doubled several times, the child having his buttocks raised upward. Also, he will be bent a little backward in order that he may have his inspiration and expiration free and also so that the nervous parts do not stretch but relax in order better to give passage to the stone when one pulls it out. It is necessary further to hold the hands of the child on top of his thigh, above his knee, spreading his thighs, in order that the work may be more surely and better done. And being thus situated, the surgeon will put his two fingers of the left hand within the rectum, the farthest forward that he can, and will press with the other hand on the lower belly, having first put a piece of linen cloth on it in order to offend and bruise less the parts thus pressed, for fear that afterward there might come inflammation and other complications, rather than by the incision. This compression is made in order to make the stone descend to the bottom of the bladder under the pubis toward the neck of the bladder and, having guided it, the surgeon must to hold it subject, for fear that it may return into the capacity of the bladder. That done, the surgeon will make an incision in the perineum, at two fingers near the seat beside the suture, with a razor with a cutting edge on both sides, of which you have had the illustration in the treatise on gangrenes. And with this all the flesh will be cut gently until one has reached the stone.

In making such an incision, it is necessary to give such good care that one does not cut the cecum because sometimes if one does not take good care in it, in attracting the stone to the neck of the bladder, the intestine bends and doubles itself. Then, when it is cut, the fecal matter comes out a part through the wound and the urine through the seat, which then forever after prevents the consolidation of the wound. This has happened to some, but also many have not failed to be well cured, because youth does things which seem to be impossible. Having made the incision, it is necessary to draw and put the stone out by such an instrument:

Little hooks proper for extracting the stone
from small children.

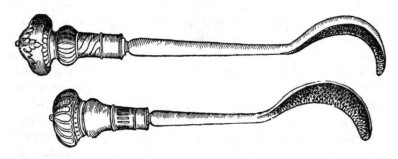

Having drawn the stone, one must apply a small cannula and hold it there some time for the reasons that we shall say hereafter and to treat it as there shall be need for preventing complications, considering the disposition and tenderness of the body. Similarly, it must not be forgotten to bind the knees together in order that the consolidation be better and more quickly made, and the rest of the cure will be made as is fitting, however, diversifying the remedies according to the temperament of the body, the tender and young being more sensitive than the old.

*On the manner of extracting the stones from men which is
called the great and high treatment. Chapter 12.*

Before the extraction of the stone the patient is to be well
purged and bled, if there is need of it, and not the next day
after he has taken medicine, because the whole body is still
stirred up by it. Further, one will be able to foment the private
parts with things which moisten and relax, in order that the stone
may be drawn out better.

It is necessary to place the patient on a firm table, the small
of his back on a cushion and under his buttocks a cloth folded
several times, and let him be leaning backward, his thighs bent
and his heels toward his buttocks. His feet must be tied
near his ankles with a strong band, three fingers wide, passing
it behind his neck two or three times, and with these his hands
will be tied against his knees, as you see by this figure:

*The figure of a man placed as is necessary when one wishes
to extract the stone from his bladder.*

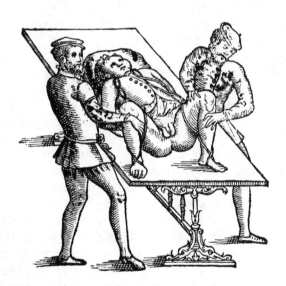

The patient being thus bound, it is necessary to have four
strong men, not fearful nor timid, that is, two to hold his arms,
and two others who will hold a knee with one hand, and with
the other the foot, so well and dextrously that he will not be
able to move his legs nor to raise his buttocks, but will remain
stable and motionless in order that the work may be better done.

The patient being thus situated, it is necessary to have a sound of silver or of iron, open on the outside and rather broad, in order that the edge of the razor can enter freely into its cavity to guide the hand of the incisor. The figure is such:

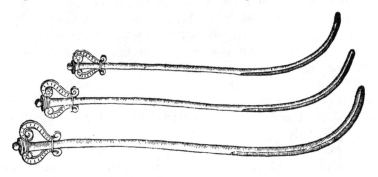

Sounds open in their exterior part.

The surgeon will pass it anointed with oil into the staff as far as the bladder and then will turn it a little toward the right side. The assistant, situated on the right hand, then with his left hand will raise the testicles upward toward the right side. That done, the surgeon will make the incision over the sound on the left side, avoiding the seam of the perineum, and likewise he will not make it too near the seat. Now the trouble which could come from making it on the seam would be that the wound could not afterward be so well reunited nor consolidated because of the callosity of this seam and because it is bloodless, and the urine passes over it, which thereafter would flow perpetually through the wound. The other trouble which could also come from making the incision too near the seat would be that one could, in drawing out the stone, break some branch of the hemorrhoid veins, which would cause a flow of blood which is staunched with difficulty in this part. Some by this error have lost their lives. Similarly, there could further be danger in drawing out the stone in that one might lacerate greatly the sphincter muscle and the body of the bladder. Therefore, the incision will be made two fingers from the seat, in the direction of the filaments, in order that afterward it may knit again better and sooner. The incision made with the razor is to be only the length of an inch because one enlarges it afterward by a crow's beak and by the dilator and especially by the stone when one draws it out. The reason why one makes the wound at the beginning so small is because that which is cut does not reunite as well and not in as brief time as that which is lacerated and torn, for the laceration is made along the direction and length of the nervous fibers. Then, after having made the incision over the sound with the razor sharp on both sides, you will put in the wound one of these silver rods, called guides (because they serve as guides to the other instruments that one wishes to introduce into the bladder), which has at its extremity a small eminence and roundness which is inserted and enters into the cavity of the sound described heretofore. The said rod is marked AA. Then it is necessary to slip above this one another which will have at its extremity a cavity and a small notch like a fork which will embrace and slip as far as the extremity of the first. The second guide is marked BB.

The figures of the guides are such, and you have them of two fashions.

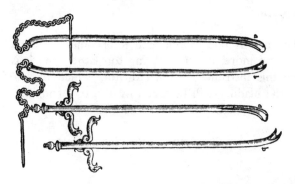

Then one will draw out the sound, and the guides will be pushed inside the body of the bladder, turning them upside down. Then one is to put the pegs in the openings in these. The others, in which there are not these pegs, are freer and are named swords by those who do such operations. Then they will be strongly compressed between the fingers of the operator. Next, between his two guides he will push with violence into the cavity of the bladder another instrument called duck's beak. Then, he will open it with both hands, turning it to right and left, here and there, with force, to lacerate and enlarge the

195

wound as much as needed in order to make passage and entry for the other instruments that must further be put in it. Yet, if it is possible to dilate the wound enough and to extract the stone by this same instrument while it is inside the bladder, this would be well done.

The figure of the duck's beak, hollow in its exterior part, is such:

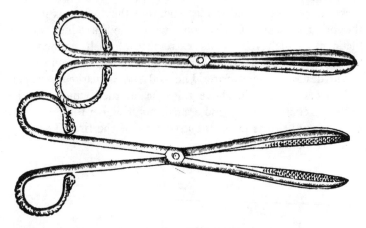

And also if one cannot, and it becomes necessary to dilate the wound more, the stone being too large, then it is necessary to use this instrument named dilator, which having been put inside the bladder will be taken by the two ends pressing them together. By that, one will dilate the wound as much as one wishes.

The figure of the closed dilator.

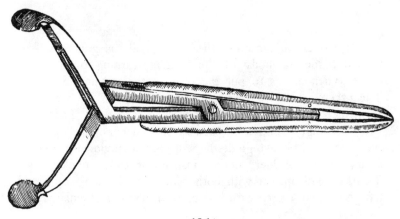

The figure of an open dilator.

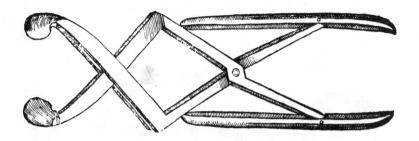

After the laceration and dilation, you will use the duck's beak written here above, or this one, which is curved.

Tenacula in form of curved duck's beak.

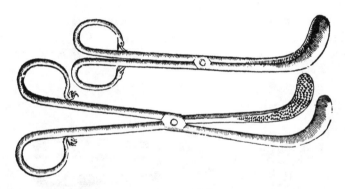

By these tenacula, the stone will be searched for, dilating the wound in order to seize it, and when the operator recognizes the stone to be between his tenaculum, it is necessary to bind the branches of it promptly and to hold it firmly, then to draw it out, not all at once, but it is necessary to turn it to one side and the other, bringing it out little by little with the greatest dexterity that one can. And in doing this, it is necessary to guard oneself from too much compressing and squeezing the stone for fear of comminuting it and breaking it into pieces. Some, in order that it may not escape from between the instruments, put two fingers inside the seat and gain control of the stone, a thing which aids greatly in drawing it out, and which I approve. The others use these two pieces called ailerons and put them beside the tenaculum, one above and the other below, then join them together, so that the stone can in no way escape, as you see by this figure:

Figure of the ailerons and of the stone taken in these with the duck's beak.

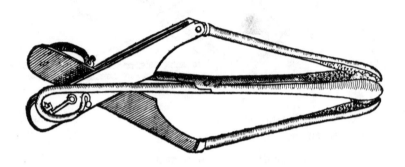

Another figure, in which at the extremity of the ailerons there is a screw to hold them better, with a piece of bent iron to compress them further; the said piece is marked a.a.

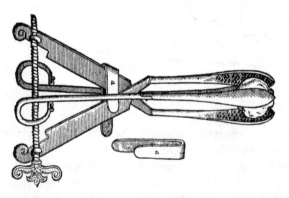

The stone drawn by the above means, it is necessary to look at it diligently to see if it is worn and polished in some place, which is done by the collision, friction, and attrition of one or several other stones. However, the most certain sign (as we have said heretofore) is the sound, which can be made at present with one of the ends of the instrument described below, which you will use as sound as well as curette.

The figure of a silver instrument, named curette, proper (after the extraction of a stone) for sounding if there are others and also for collecting and amassing the gravels, coagulated blood, and other foreign bodies which might be in the bladder, the stone drawn out.

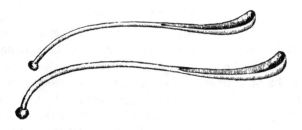

If by this one recognizes that there are other stones in the bladder, it is necessary to draw them out as before. Having thus drawn them out, it is necessary to put in the bladder the other end, which is concave in the fashion of a spoon, and to turn it to one side and another in order to take and draw out the foreign bodies that can remain in the bladder, as coagulated blood and gravel, which afterward would be the cause of formation of other stones. And where the stone would be found too large and there might be danger of breaking and lacerating the body of the bladder, wishing to draw it out, it is necessary to break it with a crow's beak such as this one:

The figure of a crow's beak for breaking the stones in the bladder.

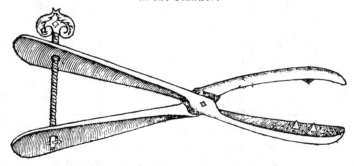

This has only three teeth, that is, two above and one below. That below will be placed so that it will enter in the middle of the two others above, and let them be in diamond point. Having broken the stone into pieces, it is necessary to take the portions out completely and to take care that no one of them remain, for there is the danger that the fragments of this one might later increase and reunite and might again make a large stone.

How it is necessary to treat the wound, the stone being drawn out. Chapter 13.

After having thus drawn out the stone and other foreign bodies, if one sees that it be necessary to make a stitch or two (leaving only the space to put a cannula), one must see that the thread be of crimson silk, rather thick and strong and waxed a little, for fear that if it were too delicate it might cut the flesh, and also might rot because of the humidity of the urine and the excrements of the wound. In doing this sewing, a rather good portion of flesh will be taken for fear that it may break and lacerate and in order that the pain caused to the patient by the sewing may not have been caused in vain and without any profit. All that done, it is necessary to put in the wound as far as into the bladder a tent of silver, cannulated and having several holes, of which you have here several descriptions:

Silver cannulae for using in the wound following the extraction of the stone, of which you have here several sorts in order to accommodate them, not the wounds to the cannulae.

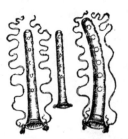 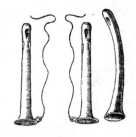

By means of these, the blood that has issued from the wound and coagulated in the bladder can be cast out and purged and also all other excrement retained in it, and it must not be held for too long a space of time for fear that nature might proceed to cast out the urine through the wound perpetually. And to the parts around it is necessary to put a repellent, such as that which follows, to repress the blood and the discharge which could be made in this because of the pain:

℞ of whites of eggs in number iii, of powder of Armenian bole, of dragon's blood, of each ℥ ii, of rose oil ℥ i, of hare's down as much as suffices. Let medicine be made in the form of honey.

On the position in which one is to place the patient after the operation. Chapter 14.

The patient will be placed in his bed, putting under him a sack full of bran or of oat straw, in order that the urine and other excrements may be soaked up in it, and it is necessary to have several of them in order to change them when there is need of it. Sometimes after the extraction blood descends in great quantity into the scrotum, so that if one does not give good and prompt care to it with resolvent, consuming, and desiccant remedies, the part turns into gangrene, which will be recognized in treating the wound. And also several days after it is necessary to make an injection through the wound into the bladder made of the liquids which follow: Take water of plantain, morel, and rose water, with a little roseate syrup. Such an injection will serve to moderate the disorder which can be in the bladder, as much from the wound as from the contusion of the instruments. The injection is to be made a little tepid and not actually cold with such a syringe:

Syringe for making injection into the bladder through the wound, after the extraction of the stone.

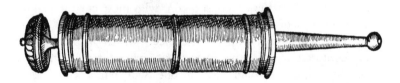

On the means by which it is necessary to remedy the retention of the urine that comes after the operation. Chapter 15.

And further, it occurs after the incision that the coagulated blood or other excrements make such obstruction in the passage of the staff that the urine cannot pass there or else does with great difficulty. Therefore, it behooves one also to put and leave a sound in the staff for some time, in order that the urine and other excrements can have issue through it.

How it is necessary to treat the wound made by the incision.
Chapter 16.

As for the wound, it is to be treated as other recent wounds, that is by digesting, cleansing, and agglutinating it, and guiding it to cicatrix. Also let the patient hold his legs crossed the one over the other in order that the union be made sooner. Let him hold to diet until the seventh or ninth day. Above all, let him avoid wine, if it is not very weak. In place of this, he will use barley water, ptisan, hippocras of water, broth, water boiled with syrup of dried roses or of Venus's-hair, and their like.

For his eating, he will use panada, grapes, little plums, pullets cooked with cold seeds, lettuce, purslane, sorrel, borage, spinach, and others similar. And if he does not have a good stomach, he will use recently freshly cleaned cassia, clysters, and other things which will be necessary for him, always according to the advice of the learned physician, if it is possible to obtain him.

On the means of curing the ulcers through which, long after the extraction of the stone, the urine still passes. Chapter 17.

Moreover, you must note here that in some men, after the stone has been drawn from them, the ulcer through which the stone has passed cannot be consolidated, and through it continually the urine issues involuntarily, whence they remain all the rest of their lives in great pain and loathsomeness, if it is not by the aid of the expert surgeon, who must cut the callosity from the lips of the wound as if it were a quite new wound. Then he will join the lips of the ulcer, which will be pinched and compressed with this instrument, named tenon, in which are three holes through which one will put needles aslant, including a rather good portion of flesh. Then you will bind the needles around the instrument, and you will apply an agglutinative medicament, as of Venice turpentine, of gum elemi, of dragon's blood, of Armenian bole. And at the end of five or six days it is necessary to remove the needles and the instrument, and you will find the ulcer almost agglutinated. Then you will finish cicatrizing it.

The figure of the tenons is such: A shows the large tenon;
B the little, which ones you will choose at your convenience.

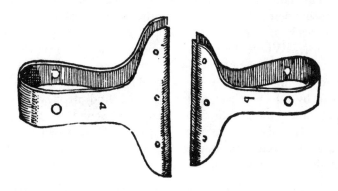

And if you did not have such instruments, you will be able in their place to use another method which I approve very much and which is easier, as follows: It is necessary to take two feather quills of the length and a little more than the ulcer may be and put them beside it and pass the stitches across these with the flesh and make the knot of the thread on these, making as many stitches as needed. By these means, the ulcer will be rejoined without breaking the flesh because of the stitches.

On the manner of drawing the stones from women.
Chapter 18.

Then, after having thus written in detail of the treatment of the stone in men by the manual operation, now I shall declare also the way in which it is necessary to aid women. First, the signs for recognizing the stones in women are such as in men but easier to be known by the sound, for the reason (as we have said here before) that they have the neck of the bladder shorter, wider, and straighter than men. Therefore, one can easily recognize if there is a stone by putting the sound in their bladder or the fingers within the neck of the womb, raising them toward the interior part of the os pubis or the penil. In doing this, one will easily find if there is stone or not, and they are to be in the same position as the men. It must be noted here that girls cannot be sounded through the neck of the womb, unless they are six to seven years old, without great violence. Therefore, in order to draw the stone from them, it is necessary to proceed as in male children, by putting the fingers within the seat. Having found the stone, one is to guide it by pressing on the lower belly with the fingers and to lead it toward the neck of the bladder, then to extract it as we have said in males. Where the girl would be old enough to permit (without violence) putting the fingers within the neck of her womb, as one does in women, the work would be done more conveniently than by putting them within the seat. And afterward, one will put inside the neck of the bladder a sound which is to be similarly hollow in its exterior part as those which have been figured heretofore, but they will not be curved but quite straight, as you see by this figure:

Sounds for making the incision in the neck of the bladder, for extracting the stones from women.

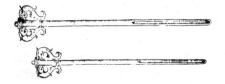

And on this, the incision will be made, and one proceeds to extract the stone, as we have said here before in males. Then it is necessary to dilate the wound with the dilator, more or less, according as there is need of it, paying heed that the neck of their bladder is short. Therefore, it must not be dilated so much for fear of lacerating the body of the bladder, for afterward patients could not hold their urine. Having dilated with laceration, the surgeon will put one or two fingers inside the neck of the womb and will press the bottom of the bladder, then will put in through this wound little hooks or tenacula and with these will take the stone, and with his two fingers which will be in the neck of the womb he will hold the stone firmly constrained and arrested from behind for fear that it may move back. Thus, it will be more easily drawn and put out.

Other practitioners operate in another fashion in the extraction of stones from females, as I have many times seen done by M. Laurent Collot, surgeon ordinary to the King, and especially by his two children, the most excellent and perfect workers in their vocation that it is possible to find in our time, and I believe that heretofore there have been few such; that is, that they do not at all put the fingers in the seat or within the neck of the womb, but content themselves with putting the guides mentioned above into the urinary tract. Thereafter they make a small incision just above and in a straight line with the orifice of the neck of the bladder, and not on the side as one does in men (in order that afterward the union may be better made). Then they pass the tenaculum, hollow in its exterior part, figured in Chapter 12, between the two guides, dilating and lacerating as much as is necessary in order to give passage to the stone, which by these means is drawn out of the bladder. The rest of the cure will be made as we have shown above in that of men. And if there occurred some ulcer in the neck of the womb by the laceration made in the extraction of the stone, one will be able to use this instrument named speculum matricis for dilating the neck of the womb in order to apply better the remedies which are necessary.

Speculum matricis.

a. shows the screw which closes and opens.

bbb. the branches which are to be of the length of eight to nine fingers.

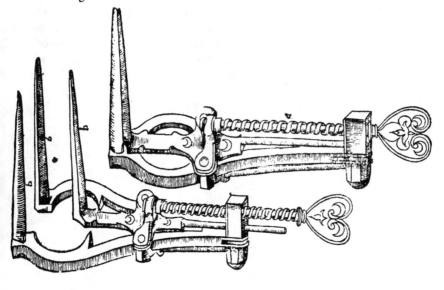

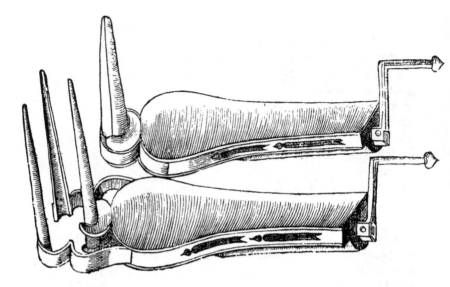

Another figure of speculum, which serves only to dilate the neck of the womb, and not to extract children from the womb, which some have falsely imagined, for they would harm there more than they could aid. The said speculums are to be of length and thickness according to the age of the women and largeness and width of the neck of their womb.

Here we shall make an end of the extraction of the stones, admonishing those from whom they will have been drawn to hold to good regimen, to the end that others may not be formed, avoiding things which greatly heat the blood and foods of heavy viscid, and glutinous juice.

End of the book of the stones.

The Tenth Book

treats of the suppression of the urine and contains 13 Chapters.

TABLE OF THE CHAPTERS OF THE TENTH BOOK.

On the Suppression

of Urine. Book X.

On the suppression of urine. Chapter 1.

Besides the causes declared heretofore of the difficulty of urinating, there are further many others which are quite necessary for the surgeon to know. Therefore, it seems to me good to write of them what I have seen and known by experience and reason, because most surgeons and others, when they see a difficulty of urinating, promptly attribute the case to come from stones, in which most often they are mistaken. As a result they go straightway and without discretion to order diuretic things, which are cause of great complications and most often of the death of the poor patients, as we shall show presently.

On the internal causes of the retention of urine. Chapter 1.*

The causes of the retention of urine are many, that is internal and external. Internal, as some coagulated blood, warts, small protuberances of flesh produced in the urinary channels, or as we have said, stones and gravels, or because the patient has had a great burning fever which has consumed the fluidity of the sanguinary mass, or by great sweats or discharge of stomach, or both together. Or for some flatulence or inflammation and abscess made in the parts dedicated to the urine or in the near and neighboring parts, as in the cecum, in which can be made an inflammation because of which the intestine, tumefied, and painful, will cause a retention of urine, for the reason that the bladder is pressed by the inflammation and swelling because of the connection and vicinity that the bladder and intestine have together. Similarly, by the fault of the liver, which one sees in the hydropic who cannot urinate; also by fault of the animal faculty, as one sees in maniacs, lethargics, apoplectics, paralytics, and in spasms. Likewise, the pituitous and other cold, heavy, and viscid humors can purge themselves from the whole body by the bladder. And this humor passing through the urinary passages sometimes produces such obstruction that it prevents the urine from passing. Also, for having re-

---

*Heading inconsistent with table of chapters.

tained the urine too long, because the bladder, being extremely full, cannot issue because the passage is contracted and narrow, in addition to the fact that the expulsive virtue cannot compress the bladder to throw out what is contained in it because of its great dilation. Therefore, there results an entire suppression of urine, which one has seen happen to many. (Recently, a young servant who was coming back from the fields carrying behind him a noble young lady, his mistress, and well accompanied and being on horseback, was taken by the wish to piss. Nevertheless, he did not dare dismount and even less to make his urine on horseback. Having arrived in this town wishing to piss, he could not at all and had very great pains and tenesmi with a general sweat, and he fell almost into syncope. Then I was sent for, and they said that it was a stone which was keeping him from pissing, and having arrived, I put a sound into his bladder. By this means, he pissed about a pint of water, and I found in it no stone and he has not since felt any.) Furthermore, from a pleurisy suppurated in the thorax, the discharge is often cast out and purged by the urines.

Digression of the author. Chapter 2.

I wish to relate to you here two marvelous examples of the providence of nature in the expulsion of things that can harm and injure it, which you will recognize by the two stories following: I have seen Monsieur Sarrest, secretary of the King, who had a pistol wound in his right arm, in which there occurred many complications and great abscesses, from which there issued a great quantity of discharge, and some days only a very little came out, and then he cast it out part by the seat and part by the urines. And when his arm discharged a great deal, one did not see in his stools nor urines any appearance of pus, and he was cured by the grace of God, and is still living at present.

Further, Germain Cheval and François Rasse, accomplished men and excellent sworn master surgeons in this town, and I have treated a gentleman named Monsieur de la Croix, who was wounded by a sword cut in his left arm, to whom a similar thing occurred; nevertheless, he died. Some held that it was impossible for the pus to make so long a road, in addition to the fact that it could not pass through the veins without spoiling the blood, and therefore, they said that such pus did not come from the arm, but from the liver or from some other part. As for me, I persisted and held for an assured thing that it was from the arm, for the reason that when from his abscesses and ulcers there issued a great quantity of pus, he did not cast out any by the lower parts. On the contrary, when they cast little or nothing, there issued a great quantity from the arm. And I said to them that it was not impossible because all our body is confluent and transpirable. Moreover, that we see by the experiment of two vessels of glass called monte-vins: one will be filled with water and the other with claret wine, and let the one be put on the other, that is the one which is filled with water on the other filled with wine, and one sees by the eye the wine mount to the top of the vessel through the water, and the water descend into the wine without mixture of the two. And if such a thing is done thus externally and openly to our sense of sight, it is also necessary to believe in our understanding that nature can make the pus pass through the veins without being mixed with the blood.

The said De la Croix dead, his body was opened and carefully searched to see if one could perceive any place from which such discharge issued, which could not be recognized. Therefore, we all concluded that death had occurred by means of the cut and not any abscess that there might be in any part within his body. Thus, it is necessary to conclude with Galen that the pus made in the interior parts and far from the kidneys and bladder can be evacuated by the urines, which by reason one can again prove. For in the excrements of the body as in the kidneys, intestines, spleen, and gall bladder, nature reserves in them some portion of blood and benign sap, proper for their nourishment, which each of these parts attracts and separates from the excrements. Further, the pure blood and the best which is in the body sent from all parts to be cast out by the staff, for the purpose of generation, passes inside the spermatic vessels, veins, and arteries which are always full of blood. Nevertheless, semen flows through without mingling in any way. Moreover, does one not see that newly delivered women cast out the milk contained in the breasts by their uterus, which also must pass inside the mammillary veins and arteries which have communication with the middle of the longitudinal muscles of the epigastrium with those of the uterus? Therefore, it must not be marveled at if the pus can be evacuated from the upper parts by the urines without being in any way mixed with the blood, for such a thing is done by the natural expulsive faculty.

And here the young surgeon will note that when we say that there are certain natural faculties, as the attractive, retentive, digestive, expulsive, assimilative, formative, visual, auditive, olfactory, gustative, sensitive, animal, vital, and natural, and others which govern our body, it must not be imagined that such faculties have understanding and reason to make their effects. For they are only instruments of our soul, which is created by GOD, and is only reasonable by the eternal providence of Him, who is incomprehensible to the human mind.

On the external causes of the retention of the urine.
Chapter 3.

The external causes are likewise many, as having bathed in cold water, or having been in the cold too long, or having excessively applied narcotic things on the region of the kidneys and used too cold foods, and other similar things. Similarly, for an interior dislocation made in the vertebrae of the loins, because of the compression of the nerves which come out from between the vertebrae, numbness is made in them, by which the expulsive faculty is enfeebled, and therefore the muscle which compresses the bladder does not permit the urine to issue.

On the prognosis of the retention of the urine.
Chapter 4.

If the urine is not evacuated as nature desires, and one is some days without urinating, the patient will die if there does not come to him fever or discharge of the stomach, or the two together, by which the urine can be consumed and evacuated by other ways than by the bladder. Some piss quite pure blood, other times mixed with urine as a water in which some piece of bloody flesh has been washed, and sometimes pure pus, or similarly mixed with the urine. The causes are many, as from too great repletion of blood, which is evacuated by period and paroxysm, as does the menstrual or hemorrhoidal flow. And to many to whom such flows have ceased, they evacuate themselves by the kidneys. Also by a type of malady resulting from congestion, or by rupture of a vein, caused by some acrid

and mordant-humor, or for having lifted too heavy a burden, or
jumped, or fallen down from a height, or having been struck
with some dry blow, or because something heavy had fallen
on the kidneys; or he had run the post and done other great
and violent exercises, and (as we have said above) because of
a stone in the kidneys having a rough surface and points or
horns; or for the imbecility of those, for having used the
venereal act immoderately, and others similar; or for having
received some wound in the parts serving the urine. Likewise,
for having used any potions, foods, and medicaments too warm,
acrid, and diuretic, and contrary in all their substance to the
parts dedicated to the urine, as cantharides and others that I
do not wish to name here.

And for these causes, there is made in the kidneys and in
the bladder so great an inflammation that it terminates most
often in abscess and suppuration and consequently ulcer, from
which the discharge is cast out by the urinary passages. And
thus we shall conclude here that the wounded parts will be
known by the signs which have preceded and are still present.
For example, if the discharge comes from the lungs, from the
liver, from the kidneys, or from the dislocated vertebrae, or
from the default of the right intestine, or from other parts, it
will be known by the position of the affected parts and by the
complications, which are fever, pain, and others which have
preceded or are still present and will demonstrate infallibly the
place whence proceeds and flows the discharge, also the quantity
and quality of the pus. For example, if it is from an ulcer
situated in the arm, as we have said when from the ulcer there
issues a quantity of pus, there will not be made emission by
the urines. On the contrary, when the ulcer remains dry, one
sees it issue by the urines or stools and in great quantity.
Similarly, if it comes from the lungs, as from an empyema or
from the liver and in abundance, it will be known because
such quantity of discharge cannot be contained in the kidneys,
besides the fact that it never resides in the bottom of the urines
but is mixed with the urines.

On the signs of ulcers in the kidneys.
Chapter 5.

The signs of ulcers of the kidneys are pain in the loins.
Further, the discharge which issues from their substance is

mixed with the urine, and one finds the sediments bloody and red. And it never issues except with the urine and always resides in the bottom of it. Further, from the ulcers of the kidneys issue sometimes small pellicles and portions of flesh and reddish filaments. Besides, it is not of as bad an odor as that which comes from the ulcer of the bladder, inasmuch as it is of nervous substance, because of which the matter cannot be as well suppurated as in the kidneys, which are fleshy.

On ulcers in the bladder, and of the signs of these.
Chapter 6.

The ulcer of the bladder can be made in the depth and capacity of it, likewise in its neck. The sign that the ulcer is in the bladder is that the patient feels perpetual pain in the depth of the pubes. And if the ulcer is in the neck, the patient feels only a little pain, except when he pisses and a little after having pissed, as we have said in the hot-pisses. The discharge which comes out of the ulcer of the bladder is very fetid, inasmuch as it is of nervous substance and as it cannot be suppurated and cooked as it is in a fleshy part, which one sees in that of the kidneys, and also that in casting it out the staff most often stiffens because of the pain that it makes passing through the urinary passage. Furthermore, one sees also within the urine little white and delicate skins and not red, or at least rarely. And one sees this discharge finally cast out of the urine and not so much mixed with the urine as when it comes from the upper parts.

On the prognosis of the ulcers in the bladder.
Chapter 7.

The ulcers of the kidneys are cured faster than those of the bladder inasmuch as they are fleshy and the bladder bloodless, membranous, nervous, and more sensitive. The ulcer which is in the depth of the bladder is incurable, or very difficult to cure, because it is nervous and because the urine which descends and remains there stings and bites, whence the ulcer always enlarges and dilates, such that it cannot be agglutinated except with great difficulty. For the urine can never be totally evacuated and the rest which is left there is warmed by the excessive heat of the bladder. And also because the bladder dilates and contracts according to the urine which it contains. That this is true we see in the suppressions of the urine a pint cast out at one stroke. When the ulcers are in the bladder and when the thighs of the patient grow lean and fall into atrophy, it is a sign of near death. If the ulcers are not quickly cured in either part, they remain incurable. If the discharge comes from the upper parts, as from the arm, as we have said, or from the lungs, from the liver, or spleen, it will be known, because such parts have first been wounded.

On the treatment of the retention of urine.
Chapter 8.

For the cure of the things which prohibit urinating, it is necessary to take indication from the malady and its cause, if it is still present. Similarly, according to the parts wounded, it is necessary to diversify the remedies, calling the physician if it is possible for you, who will prescribe for the patient the general things, and with his counsel you will put into execution what appertains to surgery.

Immediately upon seeing a difficulty of urinating, you will not run to the remedies of stones or gravels, as do often those who are not guided by method, who prescribe diuretic things, which are the cause of pernicious complications. If it were an acrid humor, or some blood caused by a contusion, or by having too much exercised the venereal act or other great and violent exercise, or having used any warm potions in which there were cantharides, or abscess and ulcers which might be in the urinary tract, or for having held his urine too long, and others similar, and if in such things one gives diuretics, one will increase the pain and the inflammation and gangrene, and consequently one will be the cause of the death of the patient. But such diuretic things could be of value when there should be some small stone or gravel, or a thick and viscid humor which has remained in the urinary passages. And likewise for having bathed in cold water or by the interior cold or undue application of narcotic things on the kidneys or to the bladder, or from an empyema, or from pituitous and cold, thick and viscid humors, which might be the cause of making obstruction in the urinary passages, and others similar, diuretics could then be of value provided further that the general things were done, and not otherwise.

Now, the diuretics can be administered in diverse fashions as follows:

To provoke the urine:

℞ of agrimony, of nettle and of pellitory having red twigs, of each m. i, of cleaned roots of asparagus ℥ iiii, of seeds of alkekengi in number xx, of seed of mallow ℥ ss, of roots of acorus ℥ i. Let all boil together in six pounds of soft water to the third, then let it be strained, of which let the patient take ℥ iiii with ℥ i of rock candy and let him drink it warm on an empty stomach three hours before food.

For the same effect:

Take ten or twelve berries of ivy and crush in white wine and give some of it to the patient to drink.

Another for the same cause:

℞ of seed of nettle pulverized ℈ i. Let it be dissolved with decoction of young chicken.
And the patient must swallow it as suddenly as he can for fear that it may adhere to the throat, because it would cause burning there.

Another:

℞ of decoction of gromwell, of Alexandrian laurel, of pellitory, of saxifrage, of root of parsley, of asparagus, of acorus, of butcher's broom, and iris, and let the patient be given to drink of it the quantity of three or four tepid ounces.

And among all, this water is excellent for provoking the urine and unstopping its passages, from whatever cause it may be:

℞ of root of water fern, of cyperus, of marshmallow graminis of parsley, of fennel, of each ℥ ii, of thicker radish cut in slices, ℥ iiii. Let them be steeped overnight in sharpest white vinegar; afterward let them boil in stream water lb. x, of saxifrage, of sea-samphire, of garance, of gromwell, of tips of mallow, of marshmallow, of each p. ii, of leaves of violets p. iii, of anagallis, of red chick-peas, of each p. i, of seed of melon, of citrul, of each ℥ ii ss, of alkekengi grains 20, of licorice ℥ i. Let all boil together to the third, in the straining infuse overnight of leaves of oriental senna lb. ss; allow once more a short boiling, in the strained expression, infuse of selected cinnamon ℈ vi. Let them be strained, once more the straining be put into a glass alembic, then add of clear Venice turpentine lb. ii, of brandy ℥ vi. Let all be stirred together very diligently, let the alembic be clayed with fire clay, let distillation be made in a bain-marie, of which you see figures.

Bain-marie

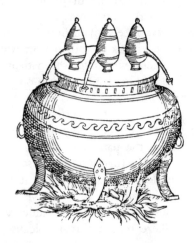

Another figure of the bain-marie.

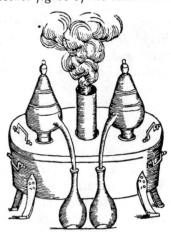

℞ of the above written distilled water ℥ ii or iii according to the operation which is preferable, four hours before eating.

Also in place of this, one can give water of radishes distilled similarly in a bain-marie and given to drink the quantity of three or four ounces with sugar, two hours before eating, and it is very proper for unstopping the urinary passages, be it of pituitous cause, gravel, or other obstruction. Baths and demi-baths, made fitly, relax, dilate, and open and soften the whole body, and on leaving these when one wishes to unstop very much, one will give diuretic things as again, for example, a half dram of theriac dissolved in water of radishes, or other similar things.

Now we shall describe some remedies for the cleansing of the ulcers of the kidneys and of the bladder. And first, the syrups of Venus's-hair, of roses drunk with hydromel, or barley water, the quantity of one ounce for each time, are good for the ulcers; also, the milk of jenny or of goat is proper for them because its serous substance cleanses them and agglutinates them because of its cheesy substance, and it nourishes because of its butyric substance. And it is to be taken, if it is possible, quite recently drawn from the animal. The patient will take a draft of it each time, with a little rose honey and a little salt, for fear it may be corrupted and turn in the stomach. Further, after having taken it, one is not to drink or eat until it is digested and has passed out of the stomach. The troches which follow are proper for cleansing ulcers of the kidneys and of the bladder:

℞ of the four greater cold seeds, of seed of white poppy, of purslane, of plantain, of quinces, of myrtles, of gum tragacanth and gum arabic, of pine nuts, of cleaned licorice, and of hulled barley, of mucilage of psyllium, of sweet almonds, of each ℥ i, of Armenian bole, of dragon's blood, of spodium, of roses, of mastic, of sealed earth, of myrrh, of each ℥ ii. According to the art let them compounded with simple oxymel, and let troches be made.

And the patient is to take a half-dram, dissolved in whey or ptisan or barley water, and others similar. Likewise, you can dissolve some in plantain water and inject some also with the syringe into the bladder. The patient, in place of wine, will drink barley water or hydromel or ptisan made with an ounce of Damascus grapes, from which one will have taken the seeds, and they will be made to boil in five pints of stream water, in a glazed pot or in a glass vial, as far as the consumption of a fourth. Then let be added to it at the end one ounce of cleaned licorice and two drams of crushed cold seeds, and then cause them to boil a little again, then pass them through the wine cloth with a quarter-pound of fine sugar and a quarter-ounce of selected cinnamon, and this will be used in place of wine. The rest of the cure will be accomplished according to the art.

On diabetes and strangury.
Chapter 9.

After having described the causes of the retention of urine and of the ulcers of the kidneys and of the bladder, I cannot pass further without declaring somewhat the causes of also casting out the urine involuntarily drop by drop, or at the very instant that the patient has drunk, which comes by the default of the retentive virtue and by a deprivation of the expulsive virtue. If the urine is cast out in great quantity, the ancients call it diabetes, and if it is cast out only drop by drop, such disposition is named strangury.

On the causes of diabetes.
Chapter 10.

The causes of diabetes are double, that is internal and external. The external are from having used intemperately too warm and diuretic things, or too immoderate great labor, and others similar. The internal causes are many, as inflammation of the liver, lungs, spleen, kidneys, bladder, or from the fault of the whole body, as by a crisis of some malady, which is terminated by flow of urines.

The causes of strangury.
Chapter 11.

The causes of strangury are also primary and antecedent, the primary from having drunk too great a quantity of cold water or having endured too great cold. The antecedents are cold humors which have flowed over the parts devoted to the urine which renders them paralytic, by means of which the muscle which restricts the bladder is relaxed and softened. Therefore, it cannot hold the bladder compressed, whence follows involuntary emission of urine.

On the signs of diabetes.
Chapter 12.

One will be able to recognize the cause to come from a warm intemperature by these signs, that is, that the patient feels a sharp and mordant pain with a great alteration and extreme thirst, joined also that he finds himself well following the use of refrigerant things and non-diuretic. On the contrary, he finds himself ill from warm things. And if the cause comes from a cold intemperature, on the contrary the pain will be small and almost insensible. And the patient will find himself ill in the use of cold things. Now, in spite of the cause of diabetes being warm, yet it is that the urine is not found tinted or red or cloudy or thick, but unsavory and white, clear, and thin, for the reason that it remains little in the liver and in the great hollow vein [vena cava] but is attracted by the intemperate warmth of the kidneys and of the bladder without any or little concoction. As for the prognosis, if such flows of urine last long, it will give the patient great weariness and he will fall into atrophy and emaciation, or wasting away of the whole body, and consequently he will die.

On the cure of diabetes.
Chapter 13.

The cure will be according to the diversity of the cause. For example, if it is by a warm intemperature the patient will be purged and bled. And it must be noted here that the four cold seeds, in spite of their being cold, are diuretic, provoking the urine. Therefore, in such disposition, it does not behoove to give any to the patient. And he will use cold and astringent foods which form thick sap, as rice, hulled barley, and their like. He will drink cold water or thick astringent wine with a good quantity of water. And on the kidneys and the parts devoted to the urine will be applied very cold and narcotic things, taking indication of the position of the kidneys, which are beneath the lumbar muscles. For this reason, you are to apply the remedies colder than if they were superficial. Then you will use oil of white poppy, of henbane, opium, of seed of purslane, of lettuce, of vinegar, of cortex of mandragora, and their like, either in liniments, cataplasms, and ointments to extinguish the foreign warmth and strengthen the affected parts. On the contrary, if the cause comes from cold, it is necessary to change the cold remedies completely, internally as well as externally, and he will use meats rather roasted than boiled.

You will content yourself, friend reader, for the present with this my work, and you will not find it out of reason if I give you here the portraits of many instruments appertaining to our art, with their names taken as much from their figure as from their usage. They are 63 in number, which I have not been able to accommodate and employ in the books that I have now brought to light; but this will be, GOD helping, for my general practice. What has moved me to have them put at the end of these books has been the fear that I had that they might not be communicated to you, being lost for many occasions to which human things are subject and also the desire that I have of serving the public, and at the same time of stimulating others to do better. For assuredly, it is a miserable thing to use invented things without adding to them, if there is need of it. This, I pray all persons to do, as much for the utility of the republic as for the acquittal of their vocation, making profit the talent that GOD has given them.

The Instruments

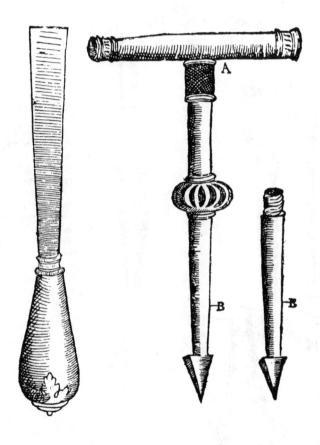

This one is called a chisel: its use is for separating the pericranium from the cranium when one expects to pierce the bone with the trepan.

Gimlet for beginning to make a small hole to place the point of the trepan.

A shows the handle.

BB the points which are inserted in the handle by a screw.

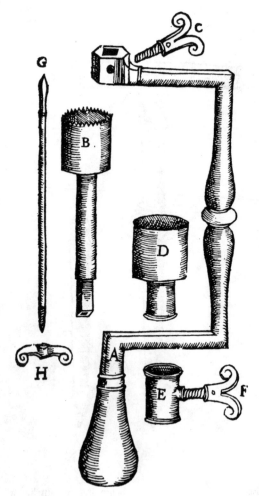

TREPAN

A the handle.
B trepan.
C the triangular point.
   holds the trepan in
   the handle.
D the hood which
   keeps the trepan
   from passing beyond
   the wish of the one
   who is trepanning.
E the band which is
   raised by such height
   as is necessary so the
   hood may give entry
   to the trepan.
F another screw which
   holds the said band
   firm.
G the triangular point.
H the ring which holds
   the said point firm.

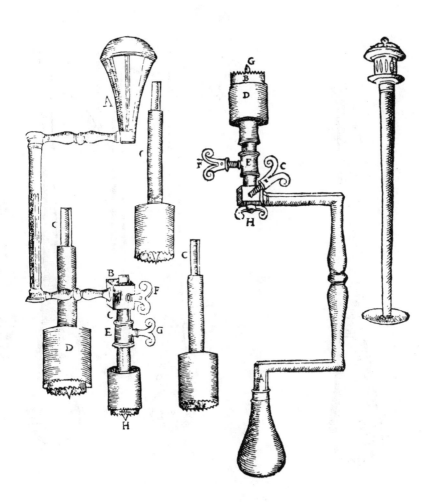

ANOTHER TREPAN
Instrument called compressor, which serves
to compress and lower the dura mater after
having trepanned, in order to make issue
forth the spread blood or sanies between
the cranium and the dura mater.

The three instruments following are saws for cutting some portion of the cranium.

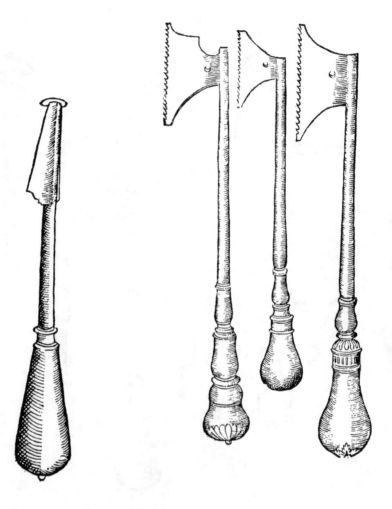

Instrument named lenticular, which cuts on one side only, for cutting any roughnesses of the bone which can sometimes remain after the trepan, at the extremity of which there is made a blunt roundness, for fear of wounding the dura mater, when one cuts the roughnesses with this.

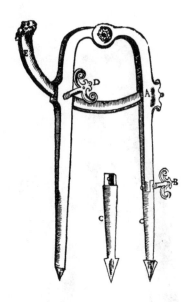

Compass for cutting the bone of the cranium.

A   The foot of the compass, which cuts the bone.
B   The small screw which holds the point.
C   Two different points, which can be inserted in the foot of the said compass.
D   The big screw, which holds a piece of iron marked E by which the compass is dilated and is closed, as is needed.

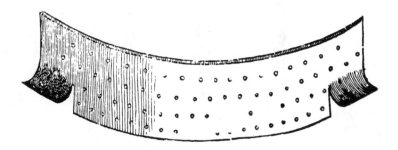

A piece of iron for supporting the compass on the head which is of curved figure with small holes, in which the leg of the compass is seated for fear it may turn here, or there.

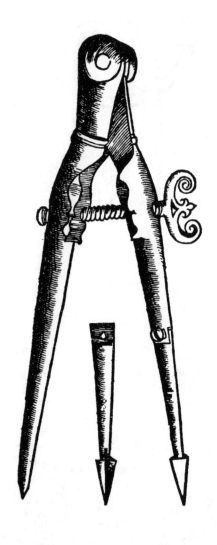

Another compass for the same use, which is dilated and closed by means of a screw.

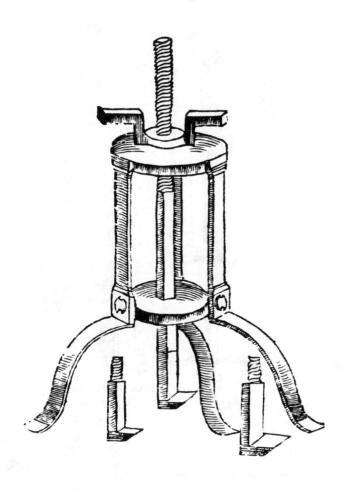

Elevator with three feet which is for drawing and elevating the bones of the head sunk in by a blow of mace of stone or otherwise: and it is of triangular figure, in order that it can be seated on all parts of the head because it is of round figure. Also, one will be able to insert into its extremity diverse points, according to need. It is raised by means of its screw.

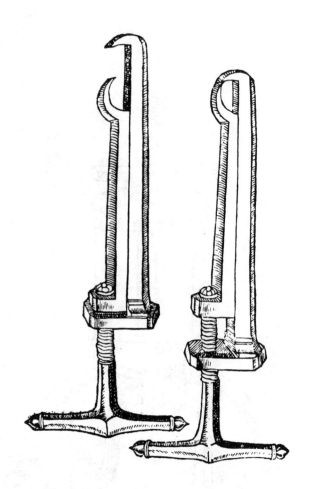

Head tenacula proper for incising and breaking the bones of the head as much and as little as one desires which is done by means of a screw.

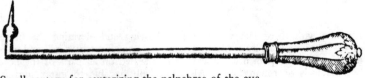

Small cautery for cauterizing the palpebrae of the eye when there is a certain hair which turns back into the eye.

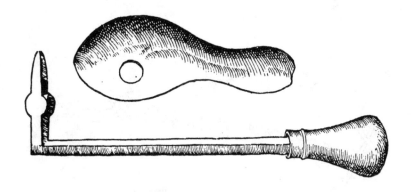

Actual cautery of triangular figure, sharp at its extremity in order that
it may do more promptly its operation, which is to cauterize a lachrymal
fistula, with a piece of iron in which there is a hole to pass the said
cautery in order that it may touch only the spot where the ill is.

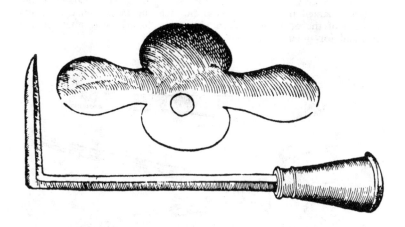

Another cautery for opening an abscess beneath the tongue, called ranula,
with a piece of iron pierced through the middle and curved to protect the
underside of the tongue.

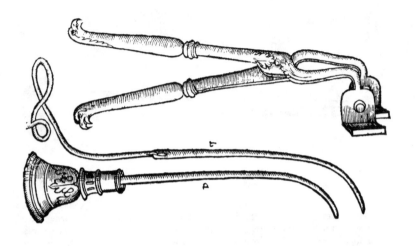

Tenacula pierced in their middle for passing a cautery marked a and a needle marked b to give a seton through the skin, which is behind the nape of the neck, in order to divert the humors which fall on the eyes, and for other dispositions of the head.

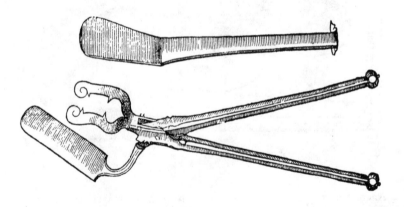

Specula oris for holding the mouth open in patients who may have some disposition in its depth.

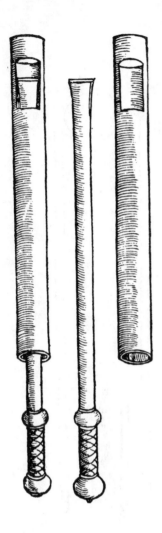

Fenestrated cannulae, with their actual cautery, for cauterizing and cutting the uvula when it is too relaxed.

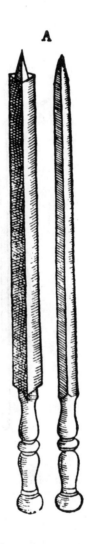

A
Another cannula with its cautery for opening any cold abscess in the gullet.

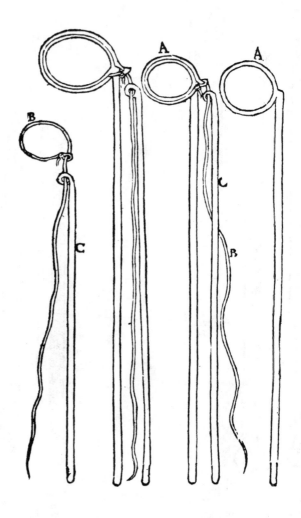

Ligatures for binding the too-relaxed uvula, provided it is whitish, long, not thick, or inflamed, which similarly can serve to bind polyps in the nose and warts in the cervix.

A Shows a ring, the upper part of which is somewhat hollow.

B A double small wire which is inserted in the upper cavity of the said ring and is tightened by means of a sliding knot.

C An iron wire, in which the said wire passes to be tightened, when one has caught the excrescent things.

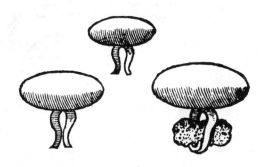

Instruments called covers, proper for covering and stopping up the
holes of the bones lost in the palate of the mouth, whether from cause of
smallpox or otherwise; without these the patients cannot pronounce their
words but speak (as is said commonly) through the nose. The said instrument will be of material of gold or of silver, and of curved figure,
and not thicker than an *écu*. To this will be attached a sponge, by which
the said instrument being inserted within the hole, the said sponge will
quickly swell by the humidity contained in the mouth, which will be the
cause of making it hold firm; and by such means the patient will pronounce his word well.

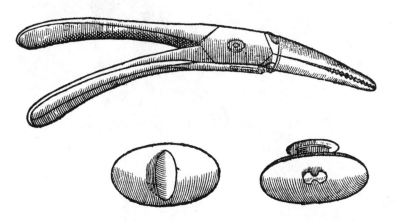

Another instrument for the same effect, without sponge, which has a
protuberance behind which turns with a little crow's beak (which you
see in this figure) when one puts it in the hole where the bone has been
lost.

233

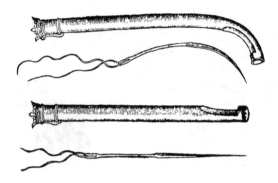

Tubes and needles for sewing wounds of the face and other parts of the body.

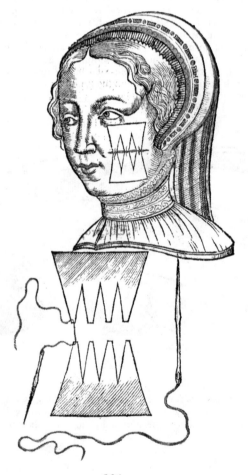

The manner of making the dry seam in order that the scars of the wounds may not remain hideous to see, which is done with two pieces of new cloth, of size that is necessary according to the wound, which are to be plastered with a certain agglutinative ointment (which I have described in my book of wounds of the head). Then they will be applied to each side of the wound and are distant from each other by one finger or about. And they will be left to dry, then sewn bringing them close one against the other.

Needle proper for sewing a varicose vein.

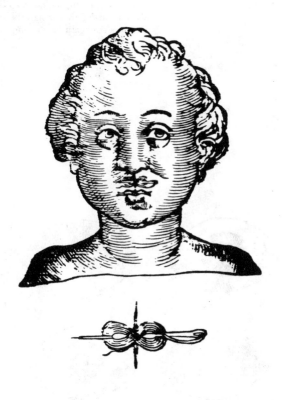

The figure of the sutures of split lips, commonly called hare's beak, and below is shown you the needle, around which the thread is wrapped as it is to be done above the lip.

235

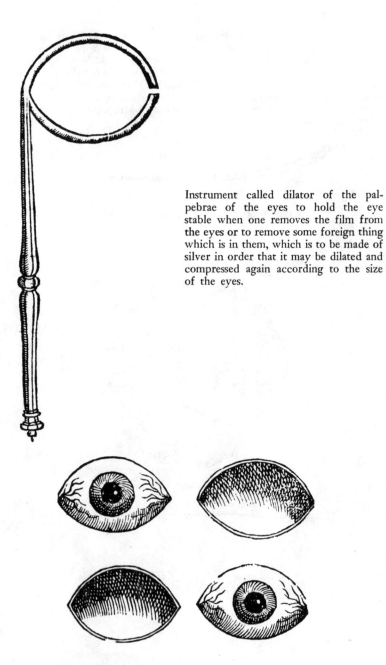

Instrument called dilator of the palpebrae of the eyes to hold the eye stable when one removes the film from the eyes or to remove some foreign thing which is in them, which is to be made of silver in order that it may be dilated and compressed again according to the size of the eyes.

Artificial eyes of which you are shown the tops and the bottoms, which will be of enameled gold and of color similar to the natural eyes.

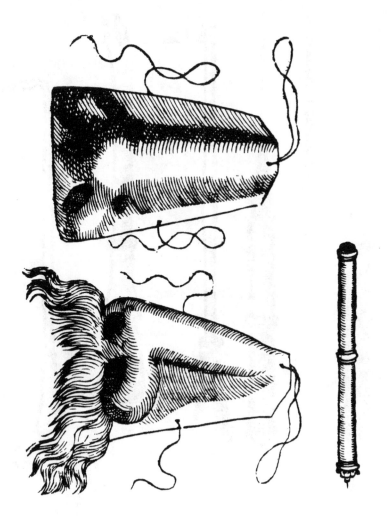

Portraits of artificial noses which are attached to a little cap, and will be painted according to the color of the one who has lost his nose.

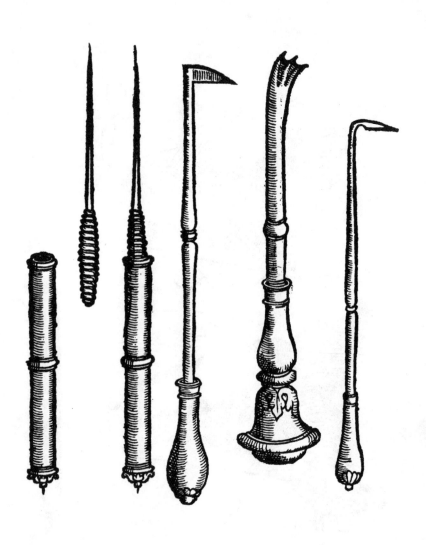

Needles proper for removing cataracts and film from the eyes.

Gum lancets, with a thruster, which is in the middle, for pushing and laying the teeth bare.

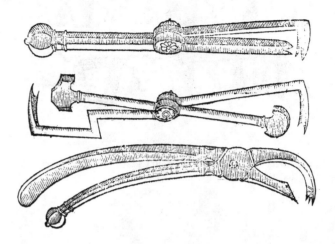

Pelicans and extraction forceps for breaking and pulling the teeth.

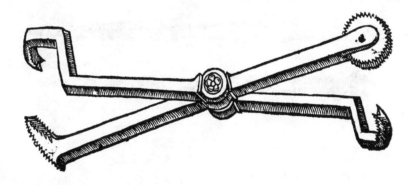

Instrument named extraction forceps (daviet), for pulling teeth.

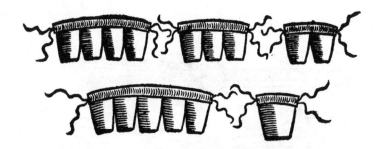

Artificial teeth made of bone which are attached by a silver wire in place of those that have been lost.

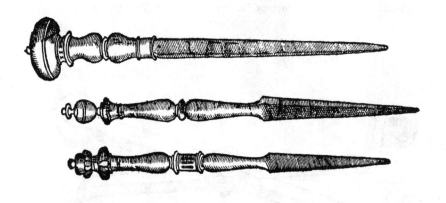

Files proper for filing the teeth.

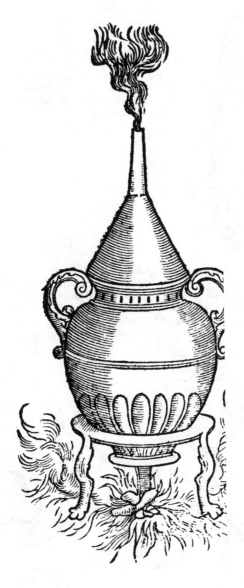

A pot with a funnel which serves it as cover, in which one will put certain drugs, of which one receives the fumes in the ears and in the neck of
the womb.

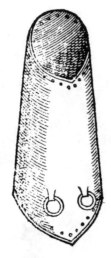

A finger stall of tin which can be attached (by means of its two small buckles) to the wrist in order to prevent the thumb from folding itself into the hand, which is done because the nerves or tendons which extend it have been cut.

The following figure shows you the portrait of a bibber made of glass, or of gold or silver, with which women suck themselves when they have too much milk in their breasts, with three little hoops with holes which serve as covering for the nipples when they are ulcered, and through the holes the milk and sanies is purged.

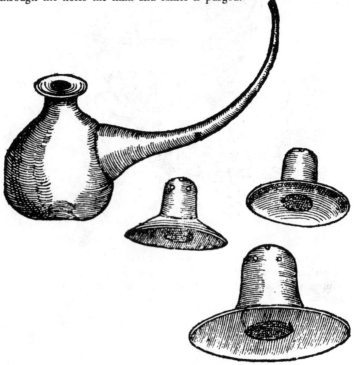

Actual cautery which has four holes for putting a small peg high or low according to whether one wishes to make it sink deep, with a flat piece of tin in the middle of this to pass the said cautery through in order that it may touch only the spot where one wishes to apply it. And the said cautery is proper to open principally the empyemas and abscesses which are within the body.

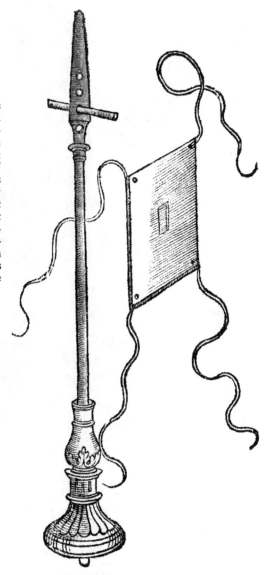

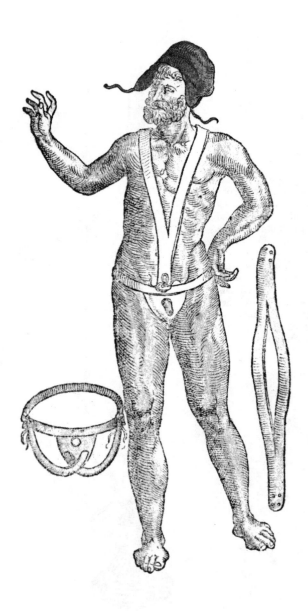

Figure which shows you a man who has a rupture on both sides and how
he is to be banded and tied with a truss to keep the intestines or omentum
from descending to the scrotum, with the figure of the truss and the
ligature called shoulder strap.

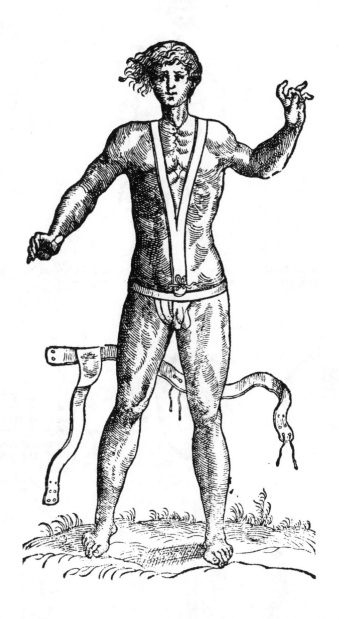

Another figure of a man who would have a rupture only on one side with a truss, in which it is necessary that there be a protuberance in the middle of the excutcheon.

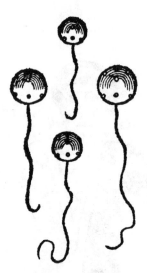

Small balls made of gold or of silver for holding an ulcer open in some part of our body, with a small cord for drawing them out.

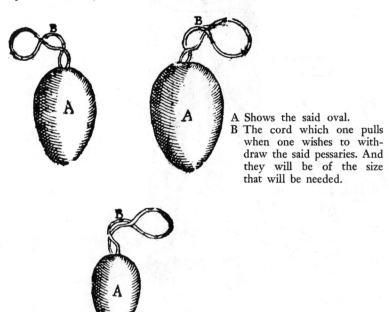

A Shows the said oval.
B The cord which one pulls when one wishes to withdraw the said pessaries. And they will be of the size that will be needed.

Pessaries in oval figure, which are to be of cork, then covered with wax, which serve to prevent the womb which is relaxed from issuing outside.

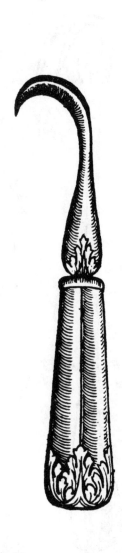

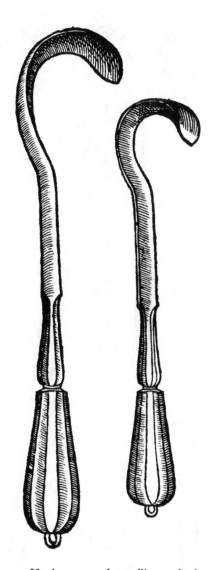

Small curved knife to split the belly and the head of a child dead in the womb in order that the excrements can be evacuated.

Hooks proper for pulling a dead child out of the belly of its mother.

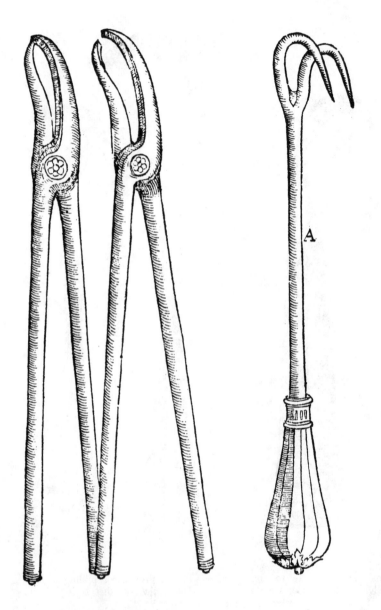

Tenacula proper to the same purpose as the preceding instrument.

A
Another hook for extracting a
mole from the womb.

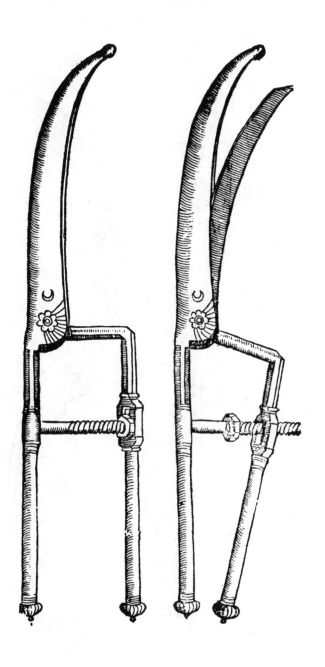

Knife proper when one wishes to cut a great quantity of flesh, which is hidden within an iron frame and is opened and closed by a screw as you can see by the eye.

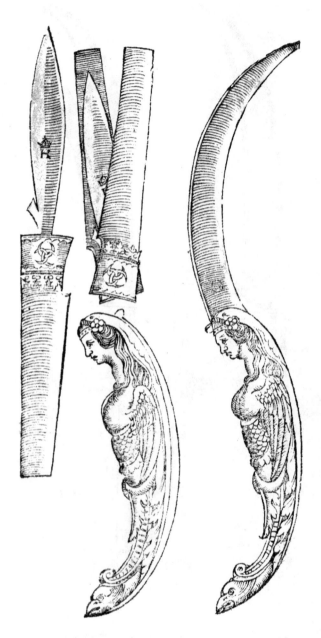

Curved and quite straight lancets proper for bleeding and opening abscesses and making other incisions.

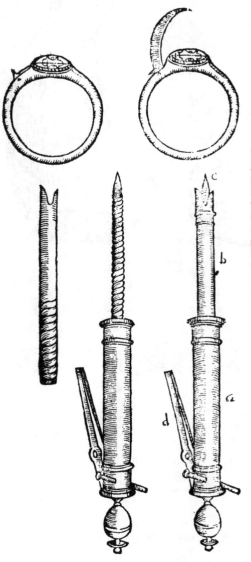

Rings in which are inserted small lancets proper for making openings in those who are timid and fearful of the instruments with pistolets for such purpose. A shows the large cannula. B another cannula, which enters into the large with a screw. C the point of the lancet which issues forth. D the spring which makes the lancet uncock.

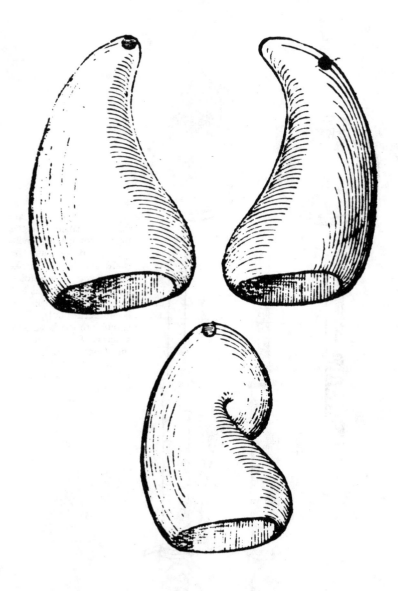

Cornets which draw without fire but by benefit of the mouth.

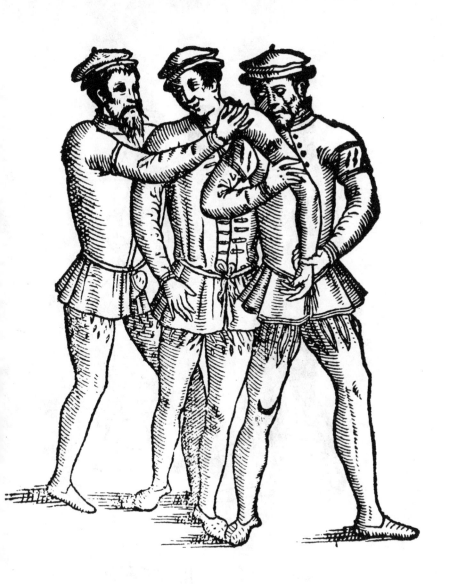

Figure which demonstrates how to reduce a complete dislocation of the left shoulder: the one in the middle is the patient, and the surgeon is the one who reduces the bone into its place, pushing it into its socket with his shoulder. And he is to be higher than the patient. The other is the assistant.

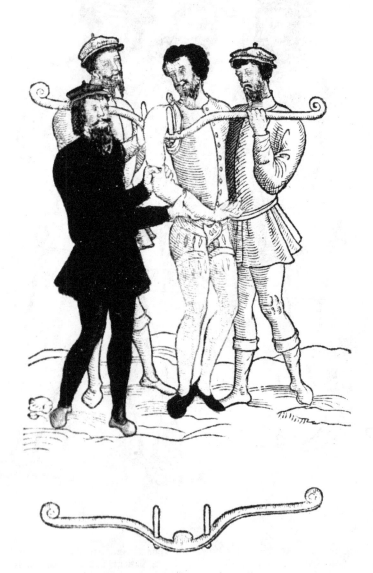

Another figure for the same purpose with a curved stick in the middle of which there is a protuberance to push the bone into its place, and two pegs preventing vacillating here and there.

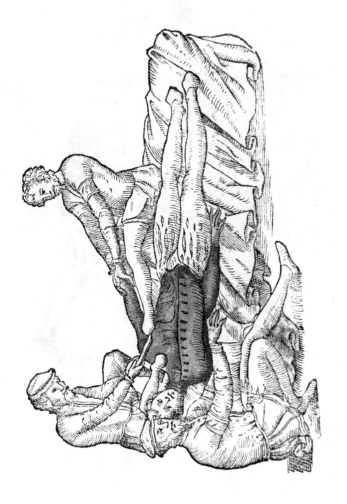

Another figure for similar disposition, which shows how to reduce the bone of the upper part of the arm by pushing it with the heel, and another which similarly raises it with a cord.

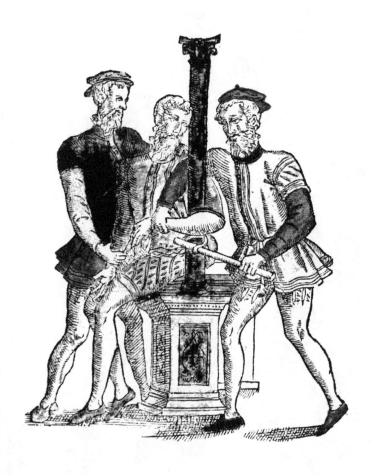

Another figure, which shows how to reduce the bone of the elbow around a pillar with a cord and a stick.

A drawer, which is proper for reducing the bone of the thigh and others.

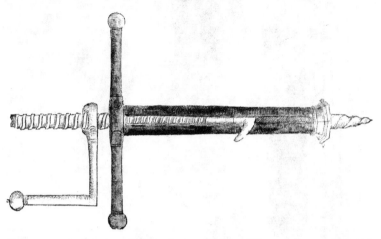

Instrument commonly called hot bath, which is of iron, and one puts inside a large block of iron likewise very hot, then one places it near a part that one expects to make sweat.

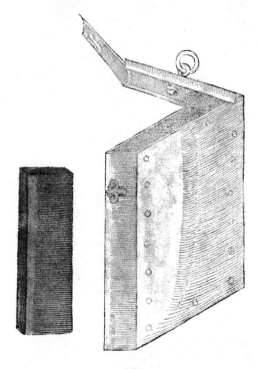

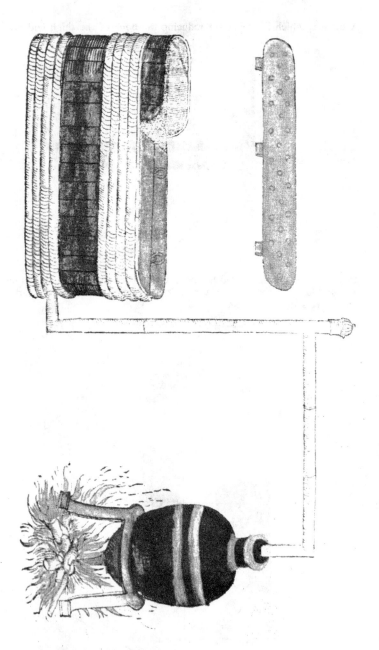

Double-bottomed tub, between which enters a vapor guided by tin pipes which comes out of a kettle, from a certain decoction for provoking sweat, which we call dry hot bath.

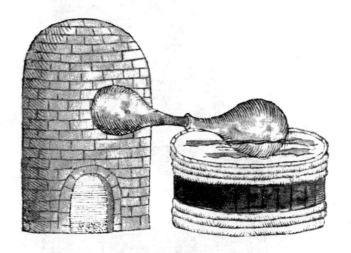

Figure of a furnace and vessel proper for distilling oil of vitriol.

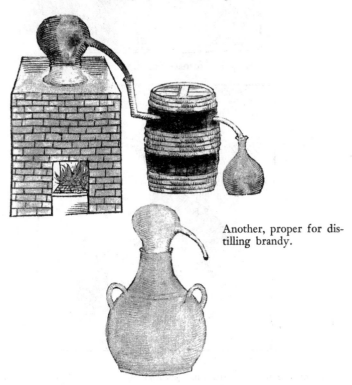

Another, proper for distilling brandy.

259

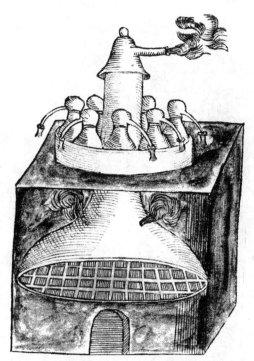

Another furnace for distilling in sand.

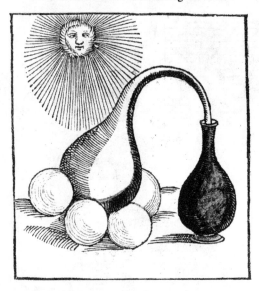

Another manner for distilling liquors by the sun's giving its warmth against great crystal balls placed under the vessel.

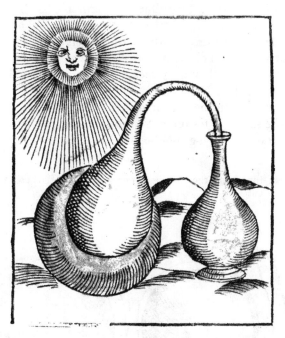

Another manner of distilling liquors, the sun striking against a burning mirror giving its reflection against the vessel. Now you will find many other furnaces and vessels in the book of Euonime Philiastre of the secret remedies, also in the book named the *Heaven of the Philosophers* and in others, with which you will be able to aid yourself as will seem good to you.

THIS which follows is to make speech possible for anyone from whom one may have cut a portion of the tongue. This invention was found by a marvelous case which happened as follows: A certain person living in the village of Ivoy le Chasteau (which is ten or twelve leagues from Bourges), who by misfortune had had his tongue out and had remained three years or more without being understandable by his speech, found himself one day in the fields with some mowers. Drinking from a rather delicate wooden bowl in their company, he was tickled by one of the said mowers while he had the bowl between his teeth, and then he uttered a few words in a way that he was understood. Then, recognizing that he had spoken thus, he took his bowl again, putting it in the same position that it was before, and again spoke so that one could well understand him with the said bowl, which was the cause that he carried it in his bosom for a long time to interpret what he wanted to say, always putting it between his teeth. Some time afterward he decided (by necessity mistress of the arts) to make an instrument of wood of such figure as follows, which he always carried hung from his neck and by means of it he did by the sound of his speech all that he wished.

The instrument here figured is to be of hard and firm wood, about the size of a teston, of figure round in circumference and flat in extent, having one of its surfaces concave the least

Instrument for aiding the speech of one a portion of whose tongue may have been cut.

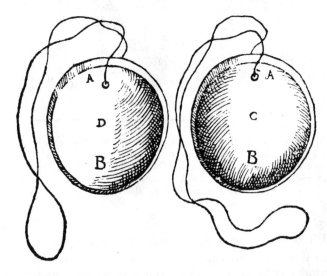

in the world, and the other convex: one of the edges bearing the thickness of a teston and the other of a half only. For example, let the edge designated by A be the thickness of a teston, and that designated by B thickness only of a half.

When it is a question of using it and using it in time, the poor mute will put the instrument in his mouth and will hold between his incisor teeth the part A, that is the part which is as thick as a teston, without anything of it appearing outside of his teeth, so that it seems that he has nothing in his mouth, and will adjust the other thinner part, that is B having only the thickness of a half teston, exactly in the place where his tongue has been cut, situating the concavity of the instrument downward and the convexity up. Doing this he will pronounce his word rather distinctly and will render himself intelligible to all those present, which is a secret unknown to us from all time but rendered well known by a fortuitous case, as we have now declared. You must not esteem this fabulous, for I assure you that, after having recovered the said instrument and the manner of using it by the aid of Monsieur le Tellier, a very learned physician residing at Bourges, I have made a trial of it in a young boy whose tongue had been inhumanly cut, who nevertheless by the benefit of this instrument pronounced his words so well that one could understand him entirely in all that he wished to say and explain. Each one, to be more certain of it, will be able to make the proof of it when he finds himself at the suitable place for doing this. Making an end here, friend reader, I shall pray you to receive this my labor with as good affection as with good will I resolve to employ all my life, my time, my work, and my study in the service of my King and to the profit of the public well-being: Which not being able to do without the grace of Him who operates all good in us and without whom we remain as mute and motionless stones, I shall entreat in this spot His majesty as maker of all things to be willing to assist and guide us in our works, if not to an exquisite perfection, at the least to some good and laudable end, according to His will.

EXTRACT OF THE PRIVILEGE

IT is permitted and granted to Master Ambroise Paré, first surgeon of the King, and sworn master at Paris, to have printed the books, treatises, portraits, and figures of anatomy as well as of the instruments of surgery and to have them placed and exposed on sale by such printers, booksellers, and merchants as will seem good to him: without other booksellers, printers, engravers of figures, dealers in colored papers, and others of whatever quality or condition they may be, and for whatever cause it may be, being able to print, portray, engrave, imitate, or counterfeit, whether in larger or smaller form, together or separately, the said books, treatises, portraits, and figures during the time and space of nine years following and consecutive, counting from the day and date that the abovesaid books, treatises, portraits, and figures of anatomy as well as instruments of surgery, will be finished printing, under penalty of confiscation of the said books and of answering for the damages and interests of the said Paré and booksellers chosen by him, with other penalty and arbitrary fine, as more fully is contained in the said letters of the privilege given on this, at Blois the third day of October, 1559, and of our reign the first.

By the King in his council.

Bourdin.

Finished printing the third day of February, 1563.